HOW TO BEAT ANGIODERMA

The Definitive Guide to Symptom Relief, Treatment, and Prevention of Similar Illnesses like Urticaria

Audrey McAllister, MD

Requests for permission to use or reproduce any part of this publication should be addressed to the publisher in writing. The publisher reserves the right to grant or deny permission at their discretion, taking into consideration factors such as the intended use, nature of the excerpt, and potential impact on the original work.

Unauthorized reproduction or distribution of copyrighted material is a violation of intellectual property rights and may result in legal consequences. Individuals or entities found to be in breach of copyright law may be subject to legal action, including but not limited to injunctions, damages, and legal fees.

It is the responsibility of all users of this publication to familiarize themselves with and abide by copyright laws and regulations. By accessing or using any part of this work, individuals agree to comply with the terms and conditions set forth by the publisher regarding copyright protection and usage rights.

TABLE OF CONTENTS

ANGIODERMA- THE OVERVIEW

Angioedema, characterized by swelling resulting from tiny blood vessels leaking fluid into the tissues, presents a challenging disorder often accompanied by breathing difficulties, necessitating immediate medical attention. The swelling associated with angioedema may persist for several days, posing discomfort and potential complications.

Although allergic causes of isolated angioedema are rare, they warrant investigation in instances where brief bouts of swelling occur under similar conditions, such as following the ingestion of specific foods or medications. Allergic reactions to food or medications often manifest as urticaria (hives) or itching alongside angioedema.

Commonly affected areas of the body include the face, lips, tongue, neck, and genital regions, although swelling can manifest anywhere. Localized swelling typically subsides within one to three days, but internal organ involvement, such as enlargement of the esophagus or stomach, may lead to chest or abdominal discomfort.

While angioedema may present with itching, tingling, or burning sensations, symptoms are generally limited to swelling-induced pain. Discomfort may escalate, particularly when swelling occurs over joints, resulting in sizable swellings that may persist for multiple days, causing prolonged discomfort and inconvenience.

SECTION 1: DEMYSTIFYING ANGIOEDEMA?

Angioedema manifests as a localized swelling beneath the skin, primarily affecting the deep dermis layer. Its acute episodes can occur in various body regions, commonly affecting the lips, mouth, eyelids, cheeks, and tongue. Additionally, it may develop in other areas such as the respiratory and gastrointestinal mucosa. Particularly concerning are instances of laryngeal or throat swelling and tongue enlargement, which can pose life-threatening risks. This condition arises from an allergic response triggering the release of histamine, causing dilation of blood vessels throughout the body.

While angioedema shares similarities with hives, which cause uncomfortable red welts on the skin's surface, it represents a more serious form of swelling.

Both hives and angioedema often stem from allergic reactions to food or medication, although pollen or insect bites can also induce angioedema. In rare cases, angioedema may signal an underlying condition such as leukemia or Hodgkin's disease.

Moreover, angioedema can arise secondary to another condition, including autoimmune diseases or infections. Some individuals experience idiopathic angioedema, where no discernible cause is identified. Hereditary angioedema presents as a rare, hereditary form of the condition that runs in families. It's important to note that angioedema differs from common types of edema (swelling) in various aspects.

Unlike edema, which typically develops gradually over days to weeks, angioedema emerges rapidly within minutes to hours. Furthermore, angioedema often exhibits asymmetry, indicating an imbalanced swelling pattern that may alter in shape. It can affect multiple body regions, including the throat, lips, face, genital region, hands, feet, and internal organs like the intestines, potentially impacting airways and causing breathing difficulties.

Most edema cases primarily affect dependent body parts, such as the lower legs and ankles, due to gravitational effects, which is not characteristic of angioedema. Moreover, while angioedema frequently accompanies hives, it can also be part of anaphylaxis, a severe allergic reaction affecting the entire body.

Angioedema is categorized into two types: mast cell-mediated angioedema and bradykinin-mediated angioedema. Mast cell-mediated angioedema is often linked with hives or other allergic response symptoms, occurring either acutely or chronically. Conversely, bradykinin-mediated angioedema, unrelated to hives, may result from certain medications like ACE inhibitors or present as hereditary or acquired conditions caused by enzyme deficiencies.

Hereditary angioedema and estrogen-dependent angioedema in females involve mutations in enzymes such as C1 esterase inhibitor or Hageman factor (Factor XII), respectively. Acquired angioedema can also occur due to a decrease in the quantity or function of these enzymes. Hence, angioedema represents a complex and multifaceted condition with various underlying causes and manifestations, necessitating tailored treatment approaches and ongoing medical supervision.

Exploring Angioedema

Angioedema, a condition marked by the swelling of deeper skin tissues, primarily manifests around sensitive areas like the eyes and mouth. The swelling can extend to the tongue and throat, posing serious challenges to breathing. While these regions are commonly affected, there are instances where swelling occurs in less common areas such as the hands, feet, and genital regions. The variability in affected areas underscores the complexity of angioedema and the diverse symptoms it presents in individuals.

The underlying mechanisms of angioedema are multifaceted, contributing to its varied manifestations. Factors such as genetic predisposition, immune system dysfunction, and allergic reactions can all play a role in triggering episodes of swelling. Consequently, individuals may experience recurring episodes of angioedema, each characterized by its unique set of symptoms and severity.

Managing angioedema episodes requires a multi-faceted approach aimed at alleviating symptoms and preventing complications. While many cases resolve spontaneously within a few days, symptomatic relief is often necessary to enhance comfort and expedite recovery. Antihistamines and steroid medications are commonly prescribed to reduce inflammation and swelling, providing relief from discomfort.

Despite the transient nature of angioedema episodes, there are instances where urgent medical attention is warranted. Breathing difficulties, in particular, necessitate immediate intervention to prevent respiratory compromise and ensure patient safety. Individuals experiencing such symptoms are advised to seek emergency medical care promptly, either by visiting the nearest emergency room or contacting emergency services for assistance.

Furthermore, understanding the triggers and underlying causes of angioedema is crucial for long-term management and prevention of recurrent episodes. Healthcare professionals play a pivotal role in this regard, conducting comprehensive evaluations to identify potential triggers and develop personalized treatment plans tailored to individual needs.

While angioedema episodes may resolve spontaneously, proactive management and timely intervention are essential for optimizing outcomes and minimizing the risk of complications. By adopting a holistic approach to care and collaborating closely with healthcare providers, individuals can effectively navigate the challenges posed by angioedema and maintain their overall well-being.

Angioedema: Recognizing its Symptoms and Signs

Angioedema swelling can manifest visibly, particularly when it affects prominent areas such as the face, notably the lips and eyelids, or when it extends to the extremities like the hands or feet. However, the implications of angioedema extend beyond mere visibility, as internal symptoms may also arise if the swelling affects internal organs, such as the colon or throat.

Of particular concern is the swelling of the throat, which can lead to severe breathing difficulties, speech impediments, or swallowing issues. This aspect of angioedema is especially critical, as throat swelling poses a significant risk of fatality, necessitating urgent medical attention to prevent potentially life-threatening airway obstruction.

In addition to the potentially life-threatening nature of throat swelling, angioedema in the intestines can cause considerable discomfort and abdominal cramps, further exacerbating the individual's distress. Moreover, angioedema may not always present in isolation; it can occur concurrently with other skin manifestations such as hives, flushing, or blotchy redness. Alternatively, it may manifest as part of an allergic reaction, indicating a broader systemic response.

Typically, angioedema resolves within a few hours to a few days, although the duration can vary significantly from person to person and even from episode to episode for a particular individual. In cases where the swelling persists or becomes severe, medical intervention may be necessary. This may involve the administration of medications to alleviate edema and manage symptoms effectively, ensuring the individual's comfort and well-being.

Angioedema poses a multifaceted challenge, ranging from visible swelling in prominent areas to potentially life-threatening complications such as throat swelling. Understanding the various manifestations and risks associated with angioedema is crucial for prompt recognition and appropriate management, underscoring the importance of timely medical intervention in severe cases.

SECTION 2: ANGIOEDEMA, URTICARIA, AND HIVES

Urticaria, commonly known as hives, manifests as itchy, raised, reddish patches on the skin, often triggered by allergens. It affects approximately 20% of the population at some point in their lives, with causes ranging from medication and illnesses to pollen and certain foods. Conversely, angioedema refers to swelling in the skin or underlying fatty tissues, distinct from hives as it affects deeper layers including the dermis, subcutaneous tissue, mucosa, and submucosal tissues.

Symptoms of hives typically manifest as itchy welts appearing on various parts of the body such as the face, chest, arms, or back. These welts, usually pink or crimson in color, can vary in size from a few millimeters to several inches. In contrast, angioedema commonly affects areas like the hands, feet, genitals, neck lining, and face, with the enlarged regions often feeling warm and uncomfortable. In severe cases, bronchospasm may occur, leading to breathing difficulties if the throat lining is affected.

Hives occur when the body's immune system reacts to an allergen by releasing histamine, causing capillaries to leak fluid into the skin, resulting in the characteristic rash. Known triggers include medications, certain foods like nuts and shellfish, infections, allergens such as pollen or dust mites, insect stings or bites, and sun exposure. Angioedema can be categorized into allergic and drug-induced types, with the former being more prevalent and typically affecting individuals allergic to substances like food, drugs, venom, pollen, or animal dander.

Treatment for acute hives often involves non-sedating antihistamines like cetirizine or fexofenadine, which mitigate the rash by blocking the effects of histamines.

Immunobiological therapy is available for severe cases of hives at specialized medical facilities. Patients with angioedema may require consultation with an allergist or immunologist, particularly if it leads to significant breathing difficulties. Identification of allergens can facilitate symptom management through over-the-counter or prescription medications and environmental avoidance strategies. Allergy testing, including skin tests and blood tests, can help identify triggers, enabling further treatments such as immunotherapy if necessary.

Causes of Angioedema: What Triggers It?

Allergic reactions can provoke histamine release into the bloodstream, triggering a cascade of physiological responses. Histamine's role involves dilating blood arteries, facilitating immune cell mobilization to injury sites, thereby causing rapid swelling, known as angioedema. Allergens such as pollen, animal dander, insect bites, and pharmaceuticals can induce this condition.

Infections and illnesses also pose a risk for angioedema development. Various diseases and disorders, including autoimmune conditions like lupus, lymphoma, and leukemia, can lead to swelling due to immune system attacks on healthy cells.

Genetic factors play a significant role in angioedema susceptibility. Hereditary angioedema, a specific subtype inherited within families, results from issues with the C1 inhibitor protein, vital for immune function and inflammation regulation. Individuals with this condition often have relatives affected by the ailment.

Certain medications can trigger drug-induced angioedema. Beta-lactam antibiotics, ACE inhibitors, and nonsteroidal anti-inflammatory drugs like aspirin and ibuprofen are commonly associated with this type of angioedema.

Environmental factors, including exposure to sunlight, water, cold, and heat, can also precipitate angioedema. These environmental variables have been shown to stimulate histamine production in the body, leading to edema in susceptible individuals.

Food intolerances can provoke allergic responses and subsequent edema in sensitive individuals. Common allergenic foods such as eggs, shellfish, milk, soy, and peanuts can induce angioedema. Additionally, lactose, monosodium glutamate (MSG), and gluten may trigger adverse reactions in some individuals.

Emotional anxiety can exacerbate angioedema symptoms. Stress-induced hormonal fluctuations, including increased cortisol, adrenaline, and histamine levels, may worsen allergic responses, leading to heightened symptoms, including angioedema, especially in individuals predisposed to allergies.

Physical exertion can also contribute to histamine release and subsequent angioedema in susceptible individuals. Intense exercise may prompt histamine generation as a protective mechanism against fatigue and depletion, particularly among individuals with a history of allergies.

Overall, awareness of these various risk factors associated with angioedema can aid in better understanding and management of this condition, promoting overall health and well-being.

How can Angioedema be Prevented?

To minimize the risk of experiencing angioedema, it is advisable to take proactive measures in various aspects of life, encompassing both lifestyle adjustments and medical considerations.

First and foremost, it's crucial to avoid exposure to known allergens, which can trigger angioedema symptoms. This entails steering clear of environments where allergens are prevalent, such as areas with high pollen levels or spaces inhabited by pets that shed dander. Additionally, certain prescription medications can contribute to angioedema, so it's essential to consult healthcare professionals about alternative treatments if you're currently taking medications that may exacerbate symptoms.

For individuals with autoimmune diseases that may induce angioedema, it's imperative to prioritize disease management. This may involve a combination of medical interventions, such as medications, physical therapy, nutritional supplements, and blood transfusions, tailored to address specific autoimmune conditions like lupus or leukemia.

Furthermore, dietary modifications can play a significant role in preventing angioedema. By identifying and avoiding foods that trigger allergic responses or sensitivities, individuals can minimize the risk of experiencing symptoms. Collaborating with healthcare providers can facilitate the development of a personalized dietary plan that ensures adequate nutrition while eliminating allergenic foods.

Effective stress management is another key component of angioedema prevention. Chronic stress can exacerbate symptoms and compromise overall well-being, making it essential to implement healthy stress management techniques. This may involve adopting relaxation practices, such as meditation or deep breathing exercises, and minimizing exposure to stressful environments or individuals.

Additionally, when engaging in physical activity, it's important to start slowly and gradually increase intensity to reduce the risk of angioedema. By gradually acclimating the body to exercise, individuals can minimize the likelihood of experiencing adverse reactions and promote overall cardiovascular health.

In summary, by taking a comprehensive approach to angioedema prevention, incorporating strategies such as allergen avoidance, disease management, medication evaluation, dietary adjustments, stress management, and gradual exercise progression, individuals can effectively mitigate the risks associated with this condition and enhance their overall quality of life.

SECTION 3: DIAGNOSING ANGIOEDEMA

During your medical consultation, the physician will inquire about your overall health and any symptoms you may be experiencing. This clinical history-taking process is paramount in unraveling the underlying causes of a person's angioedema, as it provides a comprehensive summary of the events leading up to the episodes of swelling. Keeping a detailed journal can assist in recalling these crucial details and, in certain cases, identifying recurring patterns from one episode to the next.

Given that angioedema can be associated with systemic rheumatologic illnesses, it is crucial to inform your doctor about any additional symptoms you may be experiencing, even if they seem unrelated to the angioedema itself. Moreover, it's essential to provide a comprehensive list of all medications you are currently taking, including supplements and over-the-counter drugs, as certain medications may potentially increase the likelihood of angioedema.

Following the discussion about your angioedema episodes, your healthcare practitioner may opt to conduct various laboratory tests. These tests serve to assist in differentiating between the numerous potential causes of angioedema mentioned previously. In cases where an allergic cause is suspected, particularly in instances of acute reactions, your doctor may recommend allergy skin testing or an allergen challenge, although this may not always be necessary.

Angioedema: Management and Treatment

Identification and elimination of specific triggers, whether allergens or medications, are crucial steps in halting and preventing further swelling associated with angioedema. If the condition stems from a rheumatologic disorder, addressing the underlying condition is imperative for improvement in angioedema symptoms.

In cases of severe or chronic mast-cell mediated angioedema, a comprehensive treatment approach is necessary. This may involve the use of antihistamines, steroids, and even epinephrine to alleviate swelling. Individuals experiencing facial swelling are often prescribed an EpiPen to ensure readiness for potential airway closure during an angioedema episode. Additionally, daily antihistamines may be recommended to mitigate the risk of angioedema recurrence.

If antihistamines prove ineffective in managing angioedema, alternative immunosuppressants may be considered under the guidance of a healthcare professional.

It's important to note that these medications do not address hereditary angioedema (HAE) or acquired angioedema (AAE). While various treatments exist for HAE and AAE, the most efficacious intervention involves restoring the deficient or defective C1 esterase inhibitor enzyme. This approach is essential not only in the immediate context of an angioedema episode but also in preventing its progression if episodes occur frequently enough. Recent advancements in medications include ecallantide and icatibant, which act by blocking the bradykinin pathway, offering promising avenues for treatment.

Ask Your Doctor These Questions About Angioedema Treatment

Consider the following questions to help us better understand your condition and tailor our approach to your care:

1. Have you been able to pinpoint any specific triggers that seem to coincide with your episodes of swelling?

2. In your estimation, how long do your symptoms typically last during each episode?

3. How frequently do you find yourself experiencing these episodes of swelling?

4. Apart from swelling, have you noticed any other accompanying symptoms such as stomach cramps or difficulty breathing?

5. Are you aware of any allergies that you might have, whether they be food-related or otherwise?

6. Do you find yourself frequently experiencing allergic reactions, and if so, how severe are they?

7. Have you been diagnosed with any underlying medical conditions or infections that could potentially contribute to your swelling episodes?

8. Is there a history of angioedema or swelling-related issues in your family?

9. Could you please provide a comprehensive list of all the medications you are currently taking, including dosage and frequency?

10. Have you recently introduced any new vitamins or dietary supplements into your regimen?

- 11. Have you attempted any specific treatments or interventions aimed at reducing swelling, and if so, what has been your experience with them?

SECTION 4: RECIPE IDEAS FOR MANAGING ANGIOEDEMA

MORNING MEAL IDEAS

Strawberry Breakfast Muffins

Ingredients

for 6 servings

1 cup whole wheat flour (115 g)

1 ¼ teaspoons baking powder

¼ teaspoon salt

1 cup strawberry (175 g), diced

2 eggs, room temperature

⅓ cup honey (115 g)

½ cup greek yogurt (140 g), room temperature

3 tablespoons coconut oil, melted, plus more for greasing

Directions

Preheat oven to 375°F (190°C).

In a large mixing bowl, whisk together the eggs, yogurt, honey, strawberries, and coconut oil until well combined.

Add the flour, baking powder, and salt, and fold the batter together using a rubber spatula. Stop folding once all of the dry Ingredients have disappeared into the batter.

Using a medium ice cream scoop, pour one scoop full of batter into each well of a greased muffin tin.

Bake for for 20-25 minutes, until a toothpick inserted in the center of a muffin comes out clean.

Enjoy!

Berry-Stuffed French Toast For Two

Ingredients

for 2 servings

Filling

1 cup raspberry (125 g)

1 cup blackberry (125 g)

2 tablespoons maple syrup, divided

1 tablespoon black raspberry liqueur

4 oz cream cheese (115 g), softened

French Toast

4 slices brioche bread

½ cup whole milk (120 mL)

1 large egg, beaten

2 tablespoons black raspberry liqueur

½ teaspoon salt

2 tablespoons butter

Whipped Cream

½ cup heavy cream (120 mL)

1 tablespoon maple syrup

Directions

Make the Filling: Add the raspberries, blackberries, black raspberry liqueur, and 1 tablespoon of maple syrup to a large bowl. Stir and let sit for 10 minutes for the berries to macerate.

In a medium bowl, mix together the cream cheese and remaining tablespoon of maple syrup until smooth.

Spread the Filling evenly over the 4 slices of bread. Arrange some of the berries on 2 slices of the bread and top with the other slices of bread. Press to seal the pieces together.

In a shallow dish, whisk together the milk, egg, black raspberry liqueur, and salt.

Melt the butter on a griddle or in a large skillet over medium heat. Quickly dip both sides of the bread pockets in the milk mixture, then transfer to the pan and fry on each side for about 3 minutes, until golden brown.

In a large bowl, beat the heavy cream until soft peaks form. Add the maple syrup and continue beating until the cream holds medium peaks.

Serve the stuffed French toast with a dollop of maple whipped cream and a scoop of macerated berries with their soaking liquid.

Enjoy!

Pineapple Carrot Cake Breakfast Bread

Ingredients

for 12 servings

Bread

oil, for greasing

1 ½ cups whole wheat flour (195 g)

⅓ cup organic sugar (65 g)

1 ½ teaspoons baking soda

1 ½ teaspoons baking powder

1 tablespoon ground cinnamon

1 teaspoon ground cardamom

2 teaspoons ground ginger

½ teaspoon ground cloves

½ teaspoon kosher salt

½ cup quick oat (40 g)

3 cups shredded carrots (330 g), about 3 large carrots

1 ½ cups crushed pineapple (565 g), 1 can, drained, juice reserved

3 large eggs, beaten

¼ cup butter (30 g), 1/2 stick, melted

1 cup walnuts (100 g), chopped, optional

Greek Yogurt "Frosting"

1 cup plain greek yogurt (245 g)

1 tablespoon maple syrup

Directions

Preheat the oven to 375°F (190°C). Generously grease a 9 x 4 (22 x 10 cm) loaf pan with oil.

In a large bowl, sift together the flour, sugar, baking soda, baking powder, cinnamon, cardamom, ginger, cloves, and salt. Add the oats and whisk to combine.

In a separate large bowl, combine the shredded carrots, pineapple, eggs, and melted butter. Mix well.

Add the wet Ingredients to the dry Ingredients and stir until there are no dry clumps left. Gently fold in the walnuts, if using.

Pour the batter into the prepared loaf pan and smooth the top.

Bake for 1 hour, until a toothpick inserted in the center of the bread comes out clean.

While the bread is baking, make the Greek yogurt "frosting": In a small bowl, combine the Greek yogurt, maple syrup, and 2 tablespoons of the reserved pineapple juice. Stir until well incorporated. Chill in the refrigerator until ready to use.

Remove the bread from the oven and allow to cool for 10 minutes, until safe to handle. Remove from the loaf pan and let cool completely on a wire rack.

Slice the bread and serve with a smear of frosting.

Enjoy!

Instant Oatmeal

Ingredients

for 12 servings

6 cups whole rolled oat (600 g)

½ teaspoon kosher salt

¾ cup water (175 mL), or milk, boiling

Directions

Place whole rolled oats into a large mixing bowl.

Scoop 2 cups (200 grams) of the rolled oats into a separate bowl and process in a blender or food processor until it becomes a fine powder.

Pour the blended oats into the bowl of whole rolled oats. Add salt and stir until evenly combined.

Add desired flavor additions then place the instant oatmeal mixture into an airtight container or divide into ½ cup (50 gram) single-serve portions.

When ready to eat, pour the boiling water or milk. Stir to combine and let sit for 3 minutes.

Enjoy!

Garden Vegetable Vegan Quiche

Ingredients

for 8 servings

Crust

¾ cup all purpose flour (95 g), plus more for dusting

¾ cup whole wheat flour (95 g)

½ teaspoon kosher salt

8 tablespoons vegan butter, cubed and chilled

¼ cup cold water (60 mL), plus more a needed

Filling

1 tablespoon olive oil

2 cups mushroom (150 g), thinly sliced

1 cup leek (90 g)

1 teaspoon kosher salt, divided

1 teaspoon black pepper, divided

1 cup cherry tomato (200 g)

4 cups fresh spinach (160 g)

1 package silken tofu

2 tablespoons nutritional yeast

½ teaspoon black salt, optional

½ teaspoon garlic powder

½ teaspoon paprika

¼ teaspoon ground turmeric

⅛ teaspoon cayenne pepper

Special Equipment

dried chickpea, for baking

Directions

Make the crust: In a large bowl, mix together the all-purpose flour, whole-wheat flour, and salt. Add the butter and, using your hands, work it into the flour until only pea-sized pieces remain. Continue working with your hands until the Dough has a shaggy texture.

Add the water, starting with 3 tablespoons, and mix until the Dough is moist enough to hold together. Add more water as needed, 1 tablespoon at a time. Form the Dough into a disc and wrap in plastic wrap. Refrigerate for 30-60 minutes.

Preheat the oven to 350°F (180°C).

Make the Filling: Heat the olive oil in a large skillet over medium-high heat. Once the oil is shimmering, add the mushrooms. Sauté for 3-5 minutes, until the mushrooms are beginning to brown lightly. Reduce the heat to medium and add the leeks, ½ teaspoon kosher salt, and ½ teaspoon pepper. Cook for another 3-5 minutes, until the leeks have softened slightly. Add the tomatoes and cook for 1 minute, until slightly softened. Add the spinach and sauté for 1-2 minutes, until just wilted. Remove the pan from the heat.

Lightly dust a clean surface with flour. Roll out the Dough, turning it frequently so it doesn't stick, to a 12-inch (30 cm) round, about ⅛-inch (3 mm) thick.

Gently transfer the crust to a 9-inch (22 cm) pie dish. Trim any excess Dough around the edges.

Fold the edges of Dough back underneath itself, then crimp using an index finger knuckle on one hand and the thumb and index finger on the other hand.

Crumple a piece of parchment paper, then spread it out in the center of the crust. Add the dried beans to the center and spread toward the sides of the crust--this will add weight to keep the crust from puffing up and hold up the walls while baking.

Bake the crust for 15 minutes. Carefully remove the weights by lifting out the parchment paper, then bake for 5 minutes more, until the Dough no longer looks raw.

Carefully pour the silken tofu into a fine-mesh strainer set over a bowl. Let sit for 10 minutes to allow the excess water to drain.

Add the tofu, nutritional yeast, remaining ½ teaspoon salt, remaining ½ teaspoon pepper, black salt, garlic powder, paprika, turmeric, and cayenne to a blender. Puree until smooth.

Spread half the sautéed vegetables evenly over the bottom of the crust. Pour the tofu puree over the vegetables, then add the remaining vegetables on top..

Bake for 40-45 minutes, until the center no longer jiggles and the crust is just beginning to brown.

Let the quiche cool for at least 30 minutes before slicing to allow the Filling to set.

Enjoy!

Blooming French Toast

Ingredients

for 4 servings

36 slices white sandwich bread

12 oz cream cheese (340 g), softened

⅓ cup granulated sugar (65 g), divided, plus 2 tablespoons

1 tablespoon lemon zest

1 cup whole milk (240 mL)

¾ cup heavy cream (180 mL)

½ cup light brown sugar (110 g)

3 large eggs

2 teaspoons vanilla extract

¼ teaspoon ground nutmeg

5 teaspoons ground cinnamon, divided

¼ cup strawberry preserve (80 g)

¼ cup blueberry preserves (80 g)

¼ cup raspberry preserves (80 g)

For Serving

1 cup maple syrup (335 g)

2 tablespoons powdered sugar

½ cup strawberry (75 g), sliced

½ cup blueberry (50 g)

½ cup raspberry (60 g)

Directions

Preheat the oven to 350°F (180°C).

Stack three pieces of bread on top of each other and use a rolling pin to flatten. Trim the crusts, then separate the individual slices. Repeat with the remaining bread.

In a medium bowl, combine the cream cheese, ⅓ cup (65 g) granulated sugar, and the lemon zest. Mix well, then set aside.

In a separate medium bowl, whisk together the the milk, cream, brown sugar, eggs, vanilla, nutmeg, and 2 teaspoons of cinnamon. Set aside.

Using an offset spatula, spread about 2 teaspoons of the cream cheese Filling across a slice of flattened bread. Top with 1 teaspoon of strawberry preserves and spread across the bread. Spread 11 more slices of bread with the cream cheese Filling and strawberry preserves, then repeat with the blueberry preserves and raspberry preserves.

Starting from the bottom, tightly roll up each slice of bread, then place seam-side down so they stay closed.

In a small bowl, mix together the remaining 2 tablespoons of granulated sugar and remaining 3 teaspoons of cinnamon.

Line a baking sheet with parchment paper and set a 3-inch (7.5 cm) wide bowl in the center of the pan.

Dip each roll up in the custard, allowing any excess to drip off. Arrange 12 roll ups around the bowl on the prepared baking sheet. Brush all over with custard and sprinkle with the cinnamon sugar. Repeat stacking, brushing, and sprinkling with the remaining roll ups. Remove the bowl from the center of the ring.

Bake the French toast ring for 22-25 minutes, until golden brown.

Replace the bowl in the center of the ring and fill with the maple syrup. Dust the ring with the powdered sugar. Garnish with strawberries, blueberries, and raspberries.

Enjoy!

Cheddar, Sausage, And Egg Breakfast Bake

Ingredients

for 12 servings

1 lb breakfast sausage (455 g), casings removed, crumbled

8 scallions, chopped, white\light green parts and dark green parts divided

1 red bell pepper, seeded and diced, divided

8 cups fresh spinach (320 g), packed

4 large eggs

1 teaspoon kosher salt

2 teaspoons garlic powder

2 cups whole milk (480 mL)

nonstick cooking spray, for greasing

8 cups day-old country white bread (280 g)

2 cups shredded cheddar cheese (200 g), divided

½ cup chicken stock (120 mL)

½ cup heavy cream (120 mL)

Directions

Add the breakfast sausage to a large nonstick skillet over medium heat. Cook, breaking up with a spatula until no longer pink, 7-8 minutes.

Add the white and light green scallions, ½ of the bell pepper, and ½ of the spinach. Sauté for 2 minutes, until the spinach is wilted, then add the rest of the spinach and continue cooking until wilted. Remove the pan from the heat and let cool.

In a medium bowl, whisk together the eggs, salt, and garlic powder. Add the milk and whisk to incorporate.

Grease a 9 (22 cm) x 13-inch (33 cm) glass baking dish with nonstick spray.

Add the cubed bread to the baking dish. If you don't have day-old bread, spread the cubed bread on a baking sheet and dry out in a 300°F (150°C) oven for 15-20 minutes.

Sprinkle 1 cup (100 G) of shredded cheese over the bread, then evenly spread the sausage mixture on top. Pour the egg mixture over the sausage mixture. Cover the baking dish with plastic wrap and refrigerate for at least 1 hour, or overnight.

Preheat the oven to 375°F (190°C).

In a liquid measuring cup or small bowl, combine the chicken stock and heavy cream.

Pour over the chilled bake. Sprinkle the remaining cup of cheese and remaining bell pepper over the top.

Cover with foil and bake for 45 minutes, then uncover and bake for another 15-20 minutes, until the custard is set and the cheese is golden brown. Remove from oven and let cool for 15 minutes.

Garnish with the dark green scallions, then slice and serve.

Enjoy!

Freezer-Prep Veggie Breakfast Burritos

Ingredients

for 8 burritos

olive oil, to taste

½ small white onion

1 green bell pepper, seeded and diced

1 red bell pepper, seeded and diced

1 cup cremini mushroom (75 g), sliced

kosher salt, to taste

1 cup kale (70 g), roughly chopped

8 large eggs

⅓ cup whole milk (85 g)

pepper, to taste

8 whole wheat tortillas

16 oz pinto bean (455 g)

¼ cup shredded cheddar cheese (25 g)

¼ cup shredded monterey jack cheese (25 g)

salsa, for serving

Directions

Heat a large skillet over medium heat with a drizzle of olive oil. Add the onion and cook for 3 minutes, or until translucent. Add the bell peppers and mushrooms and season with salt. Sauté for 1-2 minutes, then cover and cook for 5 minutes, until the peppers and mushrooms are softened.

Add the kale and cook until wilted. Remove the veggies from the pan and set aside. Wipe out the pan.

In a bowl, combine the eggs, milk, salt, and pepper. Whisk to combine. Set aside.

Heat another drizzle of olive oil in the clean pan. Add the eggs and cook until scrambled to your liking. Remove from the heat.

Lay a tortilla on a clean work surface. Add about ⅛ of the eggs and cooked vegetables, 2 ounces of beans, and ½ tablespoon each of the cheddar and Monterey Jack cheeses to the center. Fold in the sides of the tortilla, then roll into a burrito. Repeat with the remaining Ingredients.

Heat a clean skillet over medium-high heat. Sear the burritos on both sides, starting with the seam side, until the tortilla is brown and crisp.

Wrap the burritos individually in foil or reusable beeswax wraps. They will keep in the freezer for up to 3 weeks.

When ready to eat, unwrap a burrito and microwave for 3 minutes. Serve with salsa.

Calories: 345 Total fat: 12 grams Total carbs: 41 grams Dietary fiber: 10 grams Sugars: 4 grams Protein: 20 grams

Enjoy!

Rainbow Croissants

Ingredients

for 10 servings

⅔ cup whole milk (170 mL)

⅔ cup water (170 mL)

5 cups unbleached all-purpose flour (600 g), plus more for dusting

¼ cup granulated sugar (45 g)

1 tablespoon kosher salt

1 tablespoon instant dry yeast

3 tablespoons unsalted european-style butter, cubed, softened

5 food colorings, different colors

1 ¼ cups unsalted european-style butter (275 g), shaped into an 8X6-in (20x15-cm) rectangle, cold

1 large egg, beaten

Special Equipment

food-safe glove

Directions

In a large bowl, combine the milk and water.

On top of the liquid, add the flour, sugar, salt, yeast, and cubed butter.

Mix just until the Dough comes together, but don't overmix.

Set aside ¼ of the Dough and transfer the rest to a lightly floured surface. Knead until the flour is fully incorporated. Shape into a ball, place in a large bowl, cover with plastic wrap, and let rest at room temperature for 2 hours.

Divide the reserved quarter of Dough into 5 equal pieces. Add a few drop of different colored food coloring to each one.

Wearing food-safe gloves so you don't stain your skin, work each color into the Dough.

Shape the colored Dough into balls, place on a plate, and cover with plastic. Let rest for 2 hours at room temperature.

Transfer the large piece of rested Dough to a parchment-lined baking sheet. Shape into an 8x11-inch (20x27 cm) rectangle, cover with plastic wrap, and chill in the refrigerator overnight.

Transfer the colored Dough to another parchment-lined baking sheet. Shape into 2x3-inch (5x7 cm) rectangles, cover with plastic wrap, and chill overnight.

Transfer the plain rested Dough to a clean, lightly floured surface. Roll into a 16x8-inch (40x20 cm) rectangle. Pat the edges with a knife to straighten.

Place the butter rectangle at the center of the Dough rectangle. Fold the top and bottom of the Dough over to cover the butter, pinching the center seam and sides to seal.

Rotate 90° and roll out to a large rectangle, about 8x18 inches (20x45 cm). Flatten the edges.

Fold the top and bottom edges to meet in the center of the Dough. Fold over once more, then freeze for 30 minutes.

Roll out the Dough again to a large rectangle, about 24x8 inches (60x20 cm). Brush off any excess flour. Fold the Dough in thirds, brush again, then freeze for another 30 minutes.

Cut the chilled, colored Doughs in half lengthwise. Roll into ropes about 10 inches (25 cm) long.

Brush the ropes with water and line up together, in rainbow order or as desired. Press together. Lightly dust with flour and roll out into a rectangle roughly the same size as the plain Dough.

Brush the plain Dough with water, then lay on the colored Dough sheet on top.

Roll out into a large, 13x21-inch (33x53 cm) rectangle and about ¼-inch (6 mm) thick.

Cut the Dough into 10 triangles with bases that are about 4 inches (10 cm) wide.

Lay the Dough triangles colored side down, and starting with the wide end, gently roll up.

Place the croissants on a parchment-lined baking sheet, seam-side down. Cover with plastic wrap and let proof at room temperature for 2 hours.

Preheat the oven to 400°F (200°C).

Brush the croissants with egg wash.

Bake for 20-25 minutes, until golden brown. Let cool on a wire rack.

Enjoy!

Ricotta Chocolate Chip Stuffed French Toast With Strawberry Syrup

Ingredients

for 3 servings

For the toast

6 slices white bread

½ cup whole milk ricotta cheese (125 g)

½ cup mini chocolate chips (85 g)

2 eggs

1 tablespoon milk

sugar, pinch

For the syrup

1 cup fresh strawberry (150 g), chopped

½ cup sugar (100 g)

½ lemon, juiced

Directions

Mix the eggs with the milk and sugar.

Spread all the bread slices with ricotta cheese, and top half of the bread slices with mini chocolate chips.

Sandwich each chocolate chip half with a plain ricotta half, and drench both sides in the egg mixture.

Coat a medium heat skillet with butter, and cook the bread until slightly brown and all the egg is cooked.

To make the syrup combine all syrup Ingredients in a saucepan, and bring to a boil.

Let the liquid reduce by about a third, until the mixture is thick like a syrup.

Enjoy!

Loaded Savory Vegetable Crostata

Ingredients

for 8 servings

Crust

¾ cup all purpose flour (95 g), plus more for dusting

¾ cup whole wheat flour (95 g)

½ teaspoon kosher salt

6 tablespoons unsalted butter, cubed and chilled

3 tablespoons cold water

Filling

3 tablespoons olive oil, divided

6 cloves garlic, peeled and stems removed

1 large yellow onion, thinly sliced

1 ½ teaspoons kosher salt, divided

2 medium red potatoes, thinly sliced

⅓ cup water (80 mL)

¼ teaspoon red pepper flakes

2 rainbow swiss chards, stem and leaves separated, thinly sliced

8 oz goat cheese (225 g), room temperature

1 large egg, beaten

Directions

Make the crust: In a large bowl, mix together the all-purpose flour, whole wheat flour, and salt. Add the butter and, using a pastry cutter, work it into the flour until only pea-sized pieces remain. Add the water, starting with 3 tablespoons, and mix the Dough with your fingers until it is moist enough to hold together.

Add more water as needed, 1 tablespoon at a time. Turn the Dough onto a clean surface, form into a disc, and wrap with plastic wrap. Refrigerate for 30-60 minutes.

Preheat the oven to 375°F (190°C). Line a baking sheet with parchment paper.

While the Dough is resting, make the Filling: Add 2 tablespoons of olive oil and the garlic cloves to a large, high-walled skillet over medium heat. Cook for 3 minutes, until the garlic just begins to brown. Add the onion and ½ teaspoon of salt. Cook for 20-25 minutes, until the onion is caramelized. Remove from the pan and set aside to cool in a bowl. To the same pan, add the potatoes, ½ teaspoon of salt, and the water. Increase the heat to medium-high, cover, and cook for 3-5 minutes, until the potatoes are almost fully cooked and the water is nearly evaporated. Remove the lid and cook for 2 minutes more to completely evaporate the water. Remove potatoes from the pan and set aside to cool.

To the same pan, add the remaining tablespoon of olive oil, the red pepper flakes, and chard stems. Reduce the heat to medium and cook for 3 minutes, until the stems are softened. Add the chard leaves and remaining ½ teaspoon of salt and cook for 5 minutes, until wilted and reduced in volume by half. Remove the pan from the heat.

Remove the garlic cloves from the caramelized onions and transfer to a small bowl. Mash with the back of a fork, then add to the softened goat cheese and stir to combine.

Stir the onions into the pan with the sautéed chard.

Assemble the crostata: Roll the Dough out on a lightly floured surface into a 12-inch (30 cm) wide circle, about ⅛ inch (3 mm) thick. Transfer the Dough to the prepared baking sheet.

Spread ½ cup (110 G) of the garlic goat cheese over the center of the Dough, leaving a 2-inch (50 cm) border around the edges. Arrange half of the potatoes, slightly overlapping, over the goat cheese, then top with half of the Swiss chard and onion mixture. Repeat with remaining potatoes and chard mixture.

Fold the edges of the crust up and over the Filling to create a rustic look. Brush the crust with the beaten egg. Top with dollops of the remaining goat cheese.

Bake the crostata for 45-50 minutes, until the crust is golden brown.

Let cool for 10 minutes before slicing and serving.

Enjoy!

Cinnamon Toast Biscotti

Ingredients

for 24 biscottis

Biscotti

3 cups all purpose flour (375 g)

2 teaspoons baking powder

1 teaspoon kosher salt

½ stick unsalted butter, room temperature

1 cup granulated sugar (200 g)

1 tablespoon McCormick® Ground Cinnamon, divided, plus 2 teaspoon

2 large eggs

¼ cup whole milk (60 mL)

1 stick unsalted butter, melted

2 tablespoons turbinado sugar

Directions

Make the biscotti: Preheat the oven to 325°F (160°C). Line 2 baking sheets with parchment paper.

In a medium bowl, whisk together the flour, baking powder, and salt.

In a large bowl, combine the room temperature butter, granulated sugar, and 1 tablespoon cinnamon. Beat with an electric hand mixer on medium-high speed until fluffy, 2–3 minutes. Add the eggs, 1 at a time, beating well after each addition. Pour in the milk and beat until smooth. Add the dry Ingredientsand beat on low speed until just combined.

Divide the Dough in half and place one portion on each prepared baking sheet. Shape each into a 3-inch wide, 8½–9-inch long flat log. Refrigerate the Dough on the baking sheets for 20 minutes.

Transfer the baking sheets to the oven and bake until the logs are lightly browned around the edges, rotating the baking sheets from top to bottom and front to back halfway through, 30–35 minutes, Transfer the baking sheets to wire racks and let the logs cool for 15 minutes.

Reduce the oven temperature to 300°F (150°C).

Carefully transfer each log to a cutting board and, using a serrated knife, slice crosswise into ½-inch-thick slices. Return the slices to the baking sheets, cut-side up, spacing evenly. Brush the slices on both sides with melted butter.

In a small bowl, mix together the turbinado sugar and remaining 2 teaspoons cinnamon. Sprinkle over one side of the biscotti.

Bake until the biscotti are light brown around the edges and dry, rotating the baking sheets from top to bottom and front to back halfway through, 15–20 minutes. Transfer the baking sheets to wire racks and let the biscotti cool to room temperature before serving. Leftover biscotti will keep in an airtight container in the freezer for up to 5 days.

Enjoy!

No-Fuss Breakfast Bake

Ingredients

for 6 servings

3 tablespoons olive oil, divided

4 cups whole wheat bread (140 g), day-old, can use multigrain, or rye bread, cut into 1-inch (2 cm) cubes

1 yellow onion, thinly sliced

2 cloves garlic, finely chopped

6 cups fresh spinach (240 g), stems removed

½ lemon lemon zest

1 pinch red pepper flakes

fine sea salt, to taste

½ teaspoon fresh ground black pepper, to taste

4 eggs

4 egg whites

1 ½ cups whole milk (360 mL)

1 ½ teaspoons whole grain mustard

¼ cup grated parmesan cheese (30 g), plus 2 tbsp, divided

3 tablespoons fresh chives, finely chopped

Directions

Oil a 9x9-inch (23x23-cm) baking dish with 1 tablespoon of the olive oil and add the bread cubes in a single layer.

In a large skillet set over medium heat, add the remaining 2 tablespoons of the olive oil. Add the onions and garlic and cook until tender and starting to turn golden, 10-15 minutes.

In 2-3 batches, add the spinach and cook, tossing to wilt, 1-2 minutes.

Stir in the lemon zest and red pepper flakes and season with salt and pepper. Cook another 30 seconds then remove the pan from the heat and set aside to cool slightly.

Preheat the oven to 350°F (180°C).

In a large bowl, whisk together the eggs, egg whites, milk, and mustard. Season with salt and pepper and stir in ¼ cup (30 g) of the Parmesan.

Add the spinach mixture into the eggs. Stir in chives.

Transfer to the baking dish and mix gently to combine making sure the mixture is in an even layer. Top with remaining Parmesan.

Bake until the eggs are just set and the mixture doesn't jiggle when you gently shake the pan, 35-40 minutes.

Serve warm or at room temperature.

Enjoy!

Mixed Berry French Toast Bake

Ingredients

for 8 servings

1 loaf whole wheat bread

3 tablespoons honey

½ cup warm water (120 mL)

2 cups milk (480 mL)

6 eggs

2 teaspoons vanilla extract

2 teaspoons cinnamon

salt, to taste

½ cup blueberry (50 g)

½ cup raspberry (65 g)

½ cup blackberry (70 g)

maple syrup, to top, optional

Directions

Preheat oven to 350°F (180°C).

Slice bread into quarters. Set aside.

In a large bowl, combine honey and warm water. Whisk until the honey dissolves. Add milk, eggs, vanilla extract, cinnamon, and salt. Whisk until well-combined.

Pour the bread into a greased 9x13 (23x33 cm) baking dish. Top with the egg mixture.

Toss the bread and egg mixture together to evenly coat the bread. Let the bread soak for 20 minutes.

Add the blueberries, raspberries, and blackberries evenly on top of the bread.

Bake for 45-50 minutes until golden brown and slightly crispy around the edges and top.

NOTE: Times & temperatures may vary based on oven.

Serve with maple syrup on top (optional).

Enjoy!

Bacon Lattice Breakfast Pie

Ingredients

for 4 servings

5 eggs

1 cup whole milk (240 mL)

1 teaspoon salt

¼ teaspoon pepper

¼ cup green onion (25 g), chopped

¼ cup shredded cheddar cheese (25 g)

1 pie crust

10 slices bacon

Directions

Preheat the oven to 350°F (180°C)

Add eggs to the bowl.

In a medium-sized bowl, whisk the eggs, milk, salt, and pepper.

Add in the green onions and cheddar, and mix again.

Pour the egg mixture into the pie crust and bake for 35-40 minutes or until set.

Increase the oven temperature to 400°F (200°C).

Lay the bacon on top of the pie and weave to make a lattice top.

Bake again for 20 minutes or until bacon is crispy. Broil for crispier bacon.

Enjoy!

Homemade Cinnamon Rolls

Ingredients

for 14 servings

Dough

½ cup unsalted butter (115 g), melted

2 cups whole milk (480 mL), warm to the touch

½ cup granulated sugar (100 g)

2 ¼ teaspoons active dry yeast

5 cups flour (625 g), divided

1 teaspoon baking powder

2 teaspoons salt

Filling

¾ cup butter (170 g), softened

¾ cup light brown sugar (165 g)

2 tablespoons ground cinnamon

Frosting

4 oz cream cheese (113 g), softened

2 tablespoons butter, melted

2 tablespoons whole milk

1 teaspoon vanilla extract

1 cup powdered sugar (120 g)

Directions

Generously butter two disposable foil pie/cake pans.

In a large bowl, whisk together warm milk, melted butter, and granulated sugar. The mixture should be just warm, registering between 100-110°F (37-43°C). If it is hotter, allow to cool slightly.

Sprinkle the yeast evenly over the warm mixture and let set for 1 minute.

Add 4 cups (500g) of all-purpose flour to the milk mixture and mix with a wooden spoon until just combined.

Cover the bowl with a towel or plastic wrap and set in a warm place to rise for 1 hour.

After 1 hour, the Dough should have nearly doubled in size.

Remove the towel and add an additional ¾ cup (95g) of flour, the baking powder, and salt. Stir well, then turn out onto a well-floured surface.

Knead the Dough lightly, adding additional flour as necessary, until the Dough just loses its stickiness and does not stick to the surface.

Roll the Dough out into a large rectangle, about ½-inch (1 cm) thick. Fix corners to make sure they are sharp and even.

Spread the softened butter evenly over the Dough.

Sprinkle evenly with brown sugar and a generous sprinkling of cinnamon.

Press the mixture into the butter.

Roll up the Dough, forming a log, and pinch the seam closed. Place seam-side down. Trim off any unevenness on either end.

Cut the log in half, then divide each half into 7 evenly sized pieces. About 1½ inches (8cm) thick each.

Place 7 cinnamon rolls in each cake pan, one in the center, six around the sides. Cover with plastic wrap and place in a warm place to rise for 30 minutes.

Preheat oven to 350°F (180°C).

To prepare the frosting. In a medium-size mixing bowl, whisk together cream cheese, butter, whole milk, vanilla, and powdered sugar, until smooth.

Remove plastic wrap. Bake the cinnamon rolls in a preheated oven for 25-30 minutes, until golden brown.

While still warm, drizzle evenly with frosting.

Enjoy!

RECIPES FOR LUNCH

French Onion Soup

Ingredients

for 4 servings

4 tablespoons olive oil

2 tablespoons butter

6 cups yellow onion (900 g), thinly sliced

1 teaspoon salt

½ teaspoon sugar

3 tablespoons flour

6 cups beef stock (1.4 L)

1 cup white wine (240 mL)

½ teaspoon ground sage

1 leaf whole bay leaf

1 loaf french bread, or baguette

3 tablespoons cognac, optional

12 oz swiss cheese (340 g), grated

pepper, to taste

4 oz parmesan cheese (110 g), grated

Directions

In a large pot over medium-low heat, heat olive oil and add butter. Once the butter is melted, stir the onions and coat with oil and butter.

Cover and cook for 20 minutes, checking occasionally.

Turn up the heat to medium-high. Add ½ tsp salt and sugar. Stir and keep cooking until onions are brown and caramelized. (the bottom of the pan will develop some browning, it's very important!)

Stir in flour one tablespoon at a time and cook for about 30 seconds.

Preheat Oven To 325°F (160°C).

Add 1 cup (235 ml) of the beef broth. Use a whisk to scrape up (deglaze) the browned bits stuck on the bottom of the pan.

Add the remaining five cups of beef stock, wine, sage and bay leaf. Bring to a boil. Reduce heat and simmer, uncovered, for 40 minutes.

In the meantime, cut the french bread or baguette into ½ inch (10 mm) thick pieces. Brush with oil on both sides and bake at 325°F (160°C) for 30 minutes, flipping halfway. Once they are done, increase oven temperature to 350°F (175°C).

Add optional Ingredients.

In an oven safe bowl, pour the onion soup, Filling about ¾ of the way full. Top with a piece of baked french bread, and generously sprinkle swiss and parmesan on top.

Bake for two to three minutes or until the cheese has melted completely and become slightly golden.

Enjoy!

Meal Prep Pesto Chicken Pasta

Ingredients

for 4 servings

1 tablespoon oil

salt, to taste

1 lb large chicken breast (455 g), cooked and diced

2 cups asparagus (250 g), cut into 1 1/2-in/38-mm pieces

10 oz cherry tomatoes (285 g), halved

⅔ cup pesto (150 g)

2 cups whole wheat penne (200 g), measured dry

parsley, for garnish

Directions

Heat the oil in a large nonstick skillet. Toss in the asparagus, season with a bit of salt, and sautée until the begin to soften, about 3 minutes.

Pour on the pesto, pasta, and chicken and stir to combine.

Toss in the cherry tomatoes and give everything a stir to combine and warm through.

Distribute pasta mixture evenly between 4 tupperware containers.

Top with parsley for garnish.

Can be refrigerated up to 4 days.

Enjoy!

Elevated Hamburger Helper

Ingredients

for 4 servings

8 oz bacon (225 g), chopped

1 small yellow onion, chopped

½ cup red bell pepper (50 g), minced

1 cup shredded carrot (100 g)

2 cloves garlic, grated

1 lb lean ground beef (425 g)

kosher salt, to taste

1 tablespoon smoked paprika

2 tablespoons tomato paste, preferable double-concentrated

1 can diced tomato, petite

3 cups beef stock (720 mL)

2 cups whole milk (480 mL)

1 lb pasta shells (425 g), or short noodles of choice

2 cups shredded smoked gouda cheese (200 g)

2 cups shredded cheddar cheese (200 g)

fresh parsley, for garnish

Directions

Add the bacon to a large pot. Turn the heat to medium-high and cook until crispy, 5–7 minutes. Using a slotted spoon, transfer the bacon to a paper towel-lined plate to drain.

Discard all but 1 tablespoon of the rendered bacon fat in the pot.

Reduce the heat to medium and add the onion to the pot. Cook until softened, 5–7 minutes. Add the red bell pepper, carrots, and garlic. Cook until softened, 2–3 minutes more.

Increase the heat to medium-high and add the ground beef to the pan. Break up the beef with spatula and cook until browned, about 5 minutes. Season with salt.

Add the paprika and tomato paste. Cook until fragrant and the tomato paste turns brick-red in color, 2–3 minutes. Add the diced tomatoes, beef stock, and milk and bring to a low boil.

Once the liquid is boiling, add the pasta shells. Cover and cook for about 10 minutes, stirring occasionally, until the noodles are al dente and they have absorbed most of the liquid. NOTE: The timing will differ depending on what type of noodles you use.

Remove the pot from the heat. Stir in the Gouda and cheddar cheeses until melted. Fold in the cooked bacon.

Garnish with parsley, if desired.

Serve immediately.

Enjoy!

Uncle Pooh's Shrimp, Sausage, And Grits

Ingredients

for 6 servings

3 cups whole milk (720 mL)

3 cups heavy cream (720 mL)

1 cup white corn grit (170 g)

2 teaspoons salt, divided

1 teaspoon black pepper, divided

3 tablespoons unsalted butter

½ cup shredded cheddar cheese (50 g)

2 tablespoons vegetable oil

1 medium white onion, minced

1 yellow bell pepper, diced

1 medium red bell pepper, diced

2 cloves garlic, minced

1 lb andouille sausage (455 g), sliced

1 pinch cayenne pepper, plus more to taste

1 cup chicken stock (240 mL)

1 lb large raw shrimp (455 g), peeled and deveined

1 pinch cayenne pepper, plus more to taste

scallion, sliced, for serving

Directions

In a medium pot, stir together the milk and heavy cream over medium-high heat.

Bring to a boil.

Slowly whisk the grits into the pot. When mixture begins to bubble, reduce the heat to medium-low. Add 1 teaspoon salt and ½ teaspoon pepper.

Continue whisking the grits frequently for 10-15 minutes until mixture thickened.

Remove the grits from the heat. Add the butter and cheddar cheese, and whisk to incorporate. Set aside.

Heat the vegetable oil in a large skillet on medium-high heat.

Add the onions, peppers, and garlic. Sauté for 2 minutes until onions and peppers have softened.

Add the sausage. Cook until cooked through, about 5-7 minutes.

Slowly add the chicken stock. Stir until well-incorporated.

Add the shrimp. Cook until pink in color, about 3 minutes.

Add the cayenne, remaining teaspoon salt, and remaining ½ teaspoon black pepper. Add additional cayenne pepper, if desired.

Remove from the heat and spoon the sausage and shrimp mixture over the grits.

Sprinkle scallions on top, if desired.

Enjoy!

Pesto Pasta Freezer Prep Dinner Bake

Ingredients

for 4 servings

4 cups whole wheat pasta (800 g), cooked al dente

2 cups broccoli floret (300 g)

2 cups yellow squash (250 g), quartered

2 cups cherry tomato (400 g)

½ cup pesto (115 g)

1 cup shredded mozzarella cheese (100 g), optional

fresh basil, to serve

Directions

Preheat oven to 350°F (180°C).

Combine pasta, broccoli, yellow squash, cherry tomatoes, and pesto in freezer and oven safe baking tray.

Sprinkle mozzarella cheese on top (optional).

If freezing, cover baking tray with heavy duty foil or thick plastic wrap and store in the freezer for up to 3 months. When ready to enjoy, remove from freezer and let thaw.

Bake uncovered for 10-15 minutes.

Top with fresh basil and serve.

Enjoy!

Homemade Chicken Shawarma

Ingredients

for 4 servings

2 ½ lb boneless, skinless chicken thighs (1.1 kg), trimmed

Marinade

1 teaspoon cumin

1 teaspoon ground cardamom

1 tablespoon paprika

½ teaspoon cinnamon

1 teaspoon turmeric

1 teaspoon garlic powder

1 tablespoon sumac

¼ teaspoon cayenne

1 tablespoon kosher salt

1 teaspoon fresh ground black pepper

4 tablespoons olive oil

1 tablespoon fresh lemon juice

3 cloves garlic, sliced

White Sauce

1 cup whole milk greek yogurt (245 g)

1 tablespoon lemon juice

1 clove garlic, minced

1 teaspoon sumac

⅛ teaspoon cayenne pepper

¼ teaspoon salt

¼ teaspoon black pepper

For serving

pita bread, warmed

cucumber, sliced

tomato, sliced

pickle

Directions

Combine all marinade Ingredients in a large bowl and whisk together.

Add the chicken thighs and coat evenly.

Cover and chill for at least 1 hour and up to 12 hours

Prepare the sauce by adding all sauce Ingredients to a small bowl. Mix together and chill until ready to serve.

Adjust the oven rack about 6 inches (15 cm) from the top heat source in your oven, then preheat the broiler.

Line a baking sheet with foil and a wire rack.

Place chicken in single layer on prepared wire rack, with the smooth sides down. Broil until chicken is well browned and registers at least 165°F (74°C), about 16-20 minutes. You may need to rotate the sheet pan halfway through if your broiler heats unevenly. Remove and rest the chicken for 5 minutes before handling, and turn off the oven.

While chicken rests, warm your pitas in the still-warm oven for a few minutes.

Slice the chicken into thin strips and transfer to platter.

Serve with sliced cucumbers, tomatoes, pickles, prepared yogurt sauce, and warm pita.

Enjoy!

Black Bean & Tofu "Meat"balls

Ingredients

for 4 servings

1 package firm tofu, patted dry

15.5 oz black beans (440 g), 1 can, drained and rinsed

1 red onion, diced

1 cup spinach (40 g)

3 cloves garlic, minced

1 tablespoon tomato paste

1 dried oregano

½ teaspoon salt

½ teaspoon pepper

1 teaspoon paprika

2 cups whole wheat breadcrumbs (230 g)

1 egg

Directions

Preheat oven to 375°F (190°C).

In a blender or food processor, add tofu, black beans, onion, spinach, garlic, and tomato paste, and blend until smooth. Transfer to a large bowl.

To the bowl, add the oregano, salt, pepper, paprika, breadcrumbs, and egg. Mix well until a Dough forms.

Use your hands to form 1-inch (2-cm) balls from the black bean and tofu mixture. Place in rows on a parchment paper-lined baking sheet.

Bake for 20 minutes, or until golden, flipping halfway.

Enjoy!

Chicken Curry Naan Bowls

Ingredients

for 6 servings

Red Chicken Curry

2 tablespoons salt

1 tablespoon ground pepper

1 tablespoon ground cumin

1 tablespoon smoked paprika

1 tablespoon ground turmeric

1 tablespoon coriander

1 teaspoon ground cardamom

1 teaspoon dry mustard

1 teaspoon cayenne

½ teaspoon allspice

3 lb boneless, skinless chicken thighs (1.5 g), cut into 2 in (5 cm) cubes

5 tablespoons full-fat yogurt, divided, plus more for serving

9 cloves garlic, minced, divided

1 tablespoon fresh ginger, minced

3 tablespoons olive oil, plus more as needed

3 carrots, chopped

1 white onion, chopped

1 lb yukon gold potato (455 g), chopped

2 tablespoons tomato paste

28 oz crushed tomatoes (795 g), 1 can

2 cups chicken broth (480 mL)

2 cups basmati rice (460 g), or long-grain jasmine, cooked, for serving

1 fresh cilantro, for serving

Lime wedge, for serving

Naan Bowls

½ cup warm water (120 mL)

2 tablespoons sugar

1 tablespoon active dry yeast

4 cups all-purpose flour (500 g), plus more for dusting

1 teaspoon baking powder

1 teaspoon baking soda

1 tablespoon kosher salt, plus more to taste

1 cup full-fat yogurt (245 g)

1 cup whole milk (240 mL), room temperature

olive oil, for greasing

½ cup unsalted butter (115 g), 1 stick, melted

Directions

In a small bowl, combine the salt, pepper, cumin, smoked paprika, turmeric, coriander, cardamom, dry mustard, cayenne, and allspice. Stir to combine.

In a large bowl, add the cubed chicken thighs, 2 tablespoons of yogurt, 4 cloves of minced garlic, the ginger, and half of the spice mixture. Toss the chicken until it is fully coated. Cover the bowl with plastic wrap, and marinate in the fridge for 2 hours or overnight.

Make the naan bowls: In a liquid measuring cup, combine the warm water, sugar, and yeast. Set aside to bloom for 10 minutes.

In the meantime, mix the flour, baking powder, baking soda, and salt together in a large bowl.

To the yeast mixture, add the yogurt and milk. Stir until smooth, then pour into the dry Ingredients. Stir to combine, then dump the Dough out onto a floured surface and knead with your hands until it forms a smooth, soft ball, about 2 minutes.

Place the Dough in a clean large bowl greased with olive oil and cover with a clean kitchen towel or plastic wrap. Let rise at room temperature until doubled in size, about 2 hours.

Heat the olive oil in a large Dutch oven over medium-high heat. Working in batches to avoid overcrowding the pot, cook the marinated chicken on all sides until cooked through and browned, about 20 minutes. Drizzle in more oil, as needed, to prevent the meat from sticking to the bottom of the pot. Transfer the browned meat to a plate as it finishes cooking and set aside.

Add the carrots, onion, potatoes, remaining 5 cloves of minced garlic, and reserved spice mixture, Stir and cook until the vegetables brown slightly and start to soften, 15 minutes.

Stir in the tomato paste and cook until aromatic, about 3 minutes.

Add the crushed tomatoes and chicken broth. Stir to combine. Bring to a simmer.

Add the chicken, stir, and return to a simmer. Cover and cook for 30 minutes, or until the potatoes are tender and the chicken is cooked through.

Stir in the remaining 3 tablespoons of yogurt, then cover and keep warm.

Once the naan Dough has risen, dump onto a floured surface, and divide into 6 equal portions. Roll each portion into a ¼-inch (1 /2 cm) thick circle, approximately 10 inches (25 cm) in diameter.

Heat a large cast-iron skillet over medium-high heat. Place a disc of naan Dough in the skillet. Cook for about 2 minutes, until the Dough puffs up, then flip and cook on the other side until browned, 1 minute. Transfer the naan to a medium bowl and place another bowl on top. Repeat with the rest of the naan Dough, stacking bowls between each round. As the naan cools, they will retain the bowl shape.

Brush the naan bowls with warm melted butter.

Fill the naan bowls with the chicken curry and rice. Serve with yogurt, cilantro, and lime wedges.

Enjoy!

Garlic Herb-Crusted Roast Rack Of Lamb

Ingredients

for 8 servings

2 ½ lb rack of lamb (1.1 kg), frenched

salt, to taste

pepper, to taste

5 tablespoons olive oil, divided

8 cloves garlic, peeled and smashed

¾ cup breadcrumb (85 g)

¼ cup fresh flat-leaf parsley (10 g)

1 ½ tablespoons fresh rosemary

½ cup grated parmesan cheese (55 g)

1 ½ tablespoons whole grain dijon mustard

Directions

Preheat oven to 400°F (200°C).

Season lamb generously with salt and pepper.

Heat a cast iron over medium high heat.

To the hot pan, add in 4 tablespoons of the the olive oil, along with the lamb and garlic. Sear all sides of the lamb until browned, about 3-4 minutes. Remove browned lamb, and place cooked lamb onto a baking sheet.

Remove garlic and add to food processor with along with the breadcrumbs, parsley, parmesan, rosemary, and 1 tablespoon of olive oil. Pulse until combined. Pour onto a large plate.

Brush the top and sides of the lamb with mustard.

Coat the top and sides of the lamb with the breadcrumb mixture and roast in oven for 20-25 minutes.

Allow to rest before slicing.

Enjoy!

The Ultimate Tomato Sauce

Ingredients

for 8 servings

28 oz canned whole tomatoes (790 g), 2 cans

8 cloves garlic

¼ cup olive oil (60 mL)

2 tablespoons unsalted butter

1 large onion, finely chopped

kosher salt, to taste

pepper, to taste

2 oz anchovies (50 g), 1 tin or jar

1 teaspoon red pepper flakes

½ cup tomato paste (110 g)

½ cup dry red wine (120 mL)

1 cup water (240 mL)

1 lb spaghetti (455 g), or paste of choice, dry

1 parmesan cheese, for grating

Directions

Add the tomatoes to a deep, large bowl. Using your hands, crush the tomatoes until no large pieces remain, just a coarse tomato puree.

Peel the garlic cloves and finely chop.

Heat the olive oil and butter in a large pot over medium heat. Add the onion and garlic and season with salt and pepper. Cook, stirring occasionally, until the onion is softened but not browned, about 10 minutes.

Add the anchovies and the oil they are packed in. Cook, stirring occasionally, until dissolved into the oil, about 2 minutes.

Add the red pepper flakes and stir to combine.

Add the tomato paste and cook until it turns a dark, brick-red color, about 4 minutes (this caramelizes the sugars in the tomato, which will give a really great flavor and take the edge off that raw tomato-y taste).

Add the wine and cook for about 1 minute, just to burn off the alcohol.

Add the tomatoes and stir everything together, making sure to scrape the bottom of the pot to get all those good bits. Add water and bring it to a boil.

Reduce the heat to medium-low and cook the sauce for 1½–2 hours at a very low simmer; there should just be a few bubbles here and there. If medium-low is too high (every stove is different), reduce the heat to low. Stir every 30 minutes.

Ladle out about 2 cups of sauce: This is what is known as your "extra sauce." You'll serve it alongside the pasta or freeze it for later.

To serve, cook the spaghetti in a large pot of salted boiling water.

Drain the pasta and add it to the sauce. Serve it right out of the pot, or transfer to a serving bowl. Top with grated Parmesan cheese.

Enjoy!

Mushroom "Meat"balls

Ingredients

for 4 servings

cooking oil, or water

24 oz white mushroom (680 g), finely chopped

1 medium onion, diced

3 cloves garlic, minced

1 cup whole wheat breadcrumbs (115 g)

½ cup quick-cook oats (50 g)

¼ cup fresh parsley (10 g), chopped

2 tablespoons grated parmesan cheese

½ teaspoon dried oregano

½ teaspoon dried rosemary

½ teaspoon dried thyme

½ teaspoon salt

½ teaspoon pepper

½ teaspoon cayenne, optional

2 eggs

Directions

In a skillet over medium heat, add cooking oil or water and mushrooms. Cook down until mushrooms begin to brown, stirring occasionally.

Add the onion and cook until onions are translucent. Add the garlic and stir until fragrant. Transfer to a large bowl.

To the mushroom mixture, add breadcrumbs, oats, parsley, Parmesan, oregano, rosemary, thyme, salt, pepper, and cayenne, and stir to combine.

Add eggs and mix well.

Cover and refrigerate for at least 2 hours, or overnight.

Preheat oven to 375°F (190°C).

When ready, use your hands to form 1-inch (2-cm) balls from the mushroom mixture. Place in rows on a parchment paper-lined baking sheet.

Bake for 20 minutes, or until golden, flipping halfway.

Enjoy!

Black Bean & Tofu "Meat"balls

Ingredients

for 4 servings

1 package firm tofu, patted dry

15.5 oz black beans (440 g), 1 can, drained and rinsed

1 red onion, diced

1 cup spinach (40 g)

3 cloves garlic, minced

1 tablespoon tomato paste

1 dried oregano

½ teaspoon salt

½ teaspoon pepper

1 teaspoon paprika

2 cups whole wheat breadcrumbs (230 g)

1 egg

Directions

Preheat oven to 375°F (190°C).

In a blender or food processor, add tofu, black beans, onion, spinach, garlic, and tomato paste, and blend until smooth. Transfer to a large bowl.

To the bowl, add the oregano, salt, pepper, paprika, breadcrumbs, and egg. Mix well until a Dough forms.

Use your hands to form 1-inch (2-cm) balls from the black bean and tofu mixture. Place in rows on a parchment paper-lined baking sheet.

Bake for 20 minutes, or until golden, flipping halfway.

Enjoy!

Chickpea Garlic "Meat"balls

Ingredients

for 4 servings

water, or cooking oil

1 small onion, diced

4 cloves garlic, minced

15.5 oz chickpeas (440 g), 1 can, rinsed and drained

½ cup whole wheat breadcrumbs (60 g)

2 teaspoons fresh parsley, chopped

1 teaspoon dried oregano

½ teaspoon salt

½ teaspoon pepper

½ teaspoon red pepper flakes, optional

1 egg

Directions

Preheat oven to 375°F (190°C).

In a skillet over medium heat, add cooking oil or water and onions. Cook until onions are translucent, stirring occasionally.

Add the garlic and stir until fragrant. Transfer to a blender or food processor.

To the food processor, add the chickpeas, breadcrumbs, parsley, oregano, salt, pepper, red pepper flakes, and egg. Pulse until a Dough forms.

Use your hands to form 1-inch (2-cm) balls from the chickpea mixture. Place in rows on a parchment paper-lined baking sheet.

Bake for 20 minutes, or until golden, flipping halfway.

Enjoy!

Pizza Margherita

Ingredients

for 4 servings

4 cups bread flour (480 g)

2 ½ tablespoons kosher salt, divided

1 tablespoon sugar

2 cups warm water (470 mL)

1 ½ teaspoons active dry yeast

3 tablespoons extra virgin olive oil

28 oz whole tomatoes (795 g), san marzano or other good quality tomatoes

4 cloves garlic

1 lb fresh mozzarella cheese (455 g), sliced 1/2-inch (1 1/4 cm) thick

2 cups fresh basil (80 g)

Directions

In a large bowl combine flour, 1½ tablespoons salt, and sugar.

In a medium bowl, combine water, yeast, and 1 tablespoon of olive oil. Stir well and let rest for 2 minutes.

Add yeast mixture to flour mixture and combine using your hands or a stand mixer with a Dough hook, at least two minutes. Let Dough rest for 20 minutes, uncovered, at room temperature.

On a floured work surface, separate Dough into 4 even portions. Work each into a circular ball, then place the balls onto a baking sheet lined with wax paper. Cover with a damp towel and rest, refrigerated, for at least 4 hours.

In a blender or food processor, combine tomatoes, 2 tablespoons of olive oil, 1 tablespoon of salt, and garlic. Process until smooth.

Preheat oven to 550°F/290°C. Place a pizza stone or large cast-iron griddle on the center rack. Heat for at least 45 minutes.

On a floured work surface, use your fingertips to create a ring around the outside (your crust) of one of the risen balls of Dough. Using the pads of your fingers, gently flatten out the Dough inside the ring.

Gently lift up the Dough and let it hang off your knuckles, stretching itself out with its own weight. Slowly rotate the circle of Dough, continuing to let it stretch off your knuckles. Go all the way around the circle once, taking care not to let it hang too long in one place and stretch too thin.

Using a large spoon, spread a thin layer of sauce across the Dough, leaving room for the crust.

Evenly place three slices of mozzarella on top of the sauce, then sprinkle a handful of torn basil leaves evenly over your pizza. Or top with whatever you desire: sausage, peppers, onions... just about anything can be a pizza topping!

Carefully slide the pizza onto a floured sheet or pizza peel and place on top of your stone or griddle in the oven. Cook for 7 to 10 minutes, until the cheese is bubbly and the top of the crust is just beginning to blacken.

Remove from oven and let cool for 3-4 minutes before slicing.

Enjoy!

Classic Meatloaf

Ingredients

for 6 servings

1 tablespoon olive oil, plus more for greasing

1 large yellow onion, diced

3 cloves garlic, minced

2 tablespoons tomato paste

1 cup panko breadcrumbs (115 g)

1 cup whole milk (240 mL)

2 lb ground beef (910 g)

2 large eggs, beaten

½ cup fresh parsley (10 g), roughly chopped

1 tablespoon worcestershire sauce

½ teaspoon dried thyme

1 tablespoon kosher salt

1 teaspoon freshly ground black pepper

½ cup ketchup (120 mL)

Directions

Preheat the oven to 350°F (180°C). Line a rimmed baking sheet with foil.

Heat the olive oil in a large pan over medium-high heat. Once the oil begins to shimmer, add the onion and cook, stirring often, until softened and golden brown, about 7 minutes. Add the garlic and cook, stirring constantly, until aromatic, about 1 minute. Add the tomato paste and cook, stirring often, until the tomato paste turns deep red in color, about 2 minutes.

Remove the pan from the heat and let the onion mixture cool to room temperature.

In a large bowl, stir together the panko and milk. Add the ground beef, eggs, parsley, Worcestershire sauce, thyme, salt, pepper, and the onion mixture and use your hands to combine. Do not overmix!

Shape the beef mixture into a 10 x 5-inch loaf on the prepared baking sheet. Brush the top and sides with ketchup.

Bake the meatloaf until the top is browned and the internal temperature reaches 160°F (70°C), about 50 minutes.

Slice and serve.

Enjoy!

Greek Chicken Gyro Salad

Ingredients

for 1 serving

Tzatziki Dressing

⅔ cup plain nonfat greek yogurt (165 g)

2 tablespoons cucumber, grated, excess water squeezed out

1 tablespoon lemon juice

1 tablespoon olive oil

1 clove garlic, minced

½ teaspoon salt

Crispy Pita Chips

1 small whole wheat pita, cut into wedges

Gyro-Style Chicken

1 lemon, juiced

1 tablespoon olive oil, + 1 teaspoon, divided

1 tablespoon fresh oregano, chopped

1 lemon, zested

1 clove garlic, minced

½ teaspoon salt

¼ teaspoon ground black pepper

1 boneless, skinless chicken breast, cubed

2 cups baby spinach (80 g)

½ cup cherry tomato (100 g), halved

½ red onion, thinly sliced

½ cucumber, thinly sliced

Directions

Preheat oven to 375°F (190°C).

In a bowl, add the Greek yogurt, cucumber, lemon juice, olive oil, garlic, and salt, and stir to combine.

Place pita wedges on a baking sheet and bake until crisp, about 8 minutes.

In a bowl, add the lemon juice, 1 tablespoon olive oil, oregano, lemon zest, garlic, salt, black pepper, and chicken, and toss to coat.

Heat remaining olive oil in a pan over medium heat. Once the oil begins to shimmer, add the chicken and cook until browned, about 5 minutes.

Add the spinach, cherry tomatoes, red onion, cucumber, chicken, and pita chips together in a large bowl and drizzle with tzatziki dressing.

Enjoy!

30-Minute Burger

Ingredients

for 4 servings

Pickled Red Onions

1 ½ cups water (360 mL)

1 ½ cups apple cider vinegar (360 mL)

1 tablespoon kosher salt, plus more to taste

1 tablespoon sugar

5 whole black peppercorns

¼ teaspoon coriander seeds

1 small red onion, thinly sliced

Thousand Island Dressing

¾ cup mayonnaise (185 g)

¼ cup ketchup (60 g)

2 tablespoons pickle, finely chopped

1 clove garlic, minced

1 teaspoon white wine vinegar

Burger

2 lb ground beef (910 g), 80/20

2 teaspoons kosher salt, to taste

1 teaspoon freshly ground black pepper, to taste

1 tablespoon grapeseed oil

4 slices cheddar cheese

4 sesame buns

1 tomato, sliced, for serving

4 leaves bibb lettuce, for serving

french fry, for serving

Directions

Make the pickled red onions: In a small pot, combine the water, apple cider vinegar, salt, sugar, peppercorns, and coriander seeds, and bring to a boil over medium-high heat, stirring until the sugar dissolves.

Turn off the heat and add the sliced onion, making sure they are fully submerged. Let cool to room temperature for 30 minutes before serving.

Make the Thousand Island Dressing: In a medium bowl, whisk together the mayonnaise, ketchup, pickles, garlic, and vinegar.

In a large bowl, season the ground beef generously with salt and pepper. Use your hands to mix until evenly combined.

Divide the beef into 4 8-ounce portions and form into patties. Place on a cutting board. Use your thumb to press a divot into the center of each burger.

Heat the grapeseed oil in a cast iron or stainless steel skillet over medium-high heat until nearly smoking. Add the burger patties and cook for 3-4 minutes, without disturbing, until browned.

Use a spatula to flip the burgers over and place a slice of cheddar on each one. Cook for another

3-4 minutes, until the burgers are cooked through and cheese has melted.

Place on sesame buns and top with the pickled red onions, Thousand Island Dressing, tomato, and lettuce. Serve with French fries.

Enjoy!

Instant Pot Mac & Cheese

Ingredients

for 4 servings

1 lb dried elbow macaroni (425 g)

4 cups water (960 mL)

2 teaspoons kosher salt

3 tablespoons unsalted butter

4 cups shredded cheddar cheese

¼ cup whole milk (60 mL)

fresh parsley, for garnish - optional - chopped

Directions

Add the macaroni, water, and salt to the Instant Pot and stir to combine. Close the lid and set to pressure cook on high for 4 minutes. Once the timer goes off, set the Instant Pot to quick release.

Remove the lid, add the butter, and stir until melted. Add the cheddar cheese, then the milk, 1 tablespoon at a time, and stir until melted and creamy.

Garnish with parsley, if desired, and serve.

Enjoy!

Baked Ziti

Ingredients

for 6 servings

½ tablespoon unsalted butter

1 tablespoon olive oil

2 medium yellow onions, diced

3 cloves garlic, minced

½ teaspoon red pepper flakes

1 teaspoon dried oregano

¼ cup tomato paste (55 g)

1 can whole peeled tomato

3 teaspoons kosher salt, divided, plus more for boiling

2 teaspoons freshly ground black pepper, divided

1 package ziti or tubular pasta of choice

2 cups whole milk ricotta cheese (500 g), divided

2 cups grated parmesan cheese (250 g)

1 ½ cups shredded mozzarella cheese (150 g)

fresh basil, thinly sliced, for garnish

Directions

Preheat the oven to 400°F (200°C). Grease a 3-quart baking dish with the butter.

Heat the olive oil in a large pot or Dutch oven over medium heat. Once the oil begins to shimmer, add the onion and cook, stirring often, until softened and translucent, about 10 minutes. Add the garlic, red pepper flakes, and oregano and cook until aromatic, about 1 minute. Add the tomato paste and cook, stirring to coat the aromatics, until the tomato paste is deep brick-red, about 2 minutes.

Add the whole tomatoes and their juices, using a potato masher or your hands to crush them into the sauce. Add 2 teaspoons of salt and 1 teaspoon of pepper and stir to combine. Bring the sauce to a boil, then reduce the heat to low and simmer until thickened, 20 minutes.

Add 1 cup of ricotta, the Parmesan, remaining teaspoon of salt, and remaining teaspoon of pepper to a medium bowl and stir to combine.

Reserve 2 cups of tomato sauce in a bowl, then add the ricotta-Parmesan mixture to the remaining tomato sauce in the pot and stir to combine.

Bring a large pot of salted water to a boil over high heat. Add the pasta and cook until 2 minutes shy of al dente. Drain the pasta in a colander.

Add the drained pasta tomato-ricotta sauce and stir until well coated.

Add half of the pasta to the prepared baking dish. Cover with 1 cup of the reserved tomato sauce, ¾ cup of the mozzarella, and ½ cup of the remaining ricotta. Add the remaining pasta, then repeat with the remaining cup of tomato sauce, ¾ cup of mozzarella, and ½ cup of ricotta.

Bake until the mozzarella is golden brown and the tomato sauce is bubbling, 25–30 minutes.

Garnish with the basil before serving.

Enjoy!

Peanut Butter & Jelly Spiders

Ingredients

for 1 spider

2 slices whole grain bread

nut butter, to taste

jelly, to taste

8 pretzel sticks

2 raisins

Directions

Using the lid of a wide mouth mason jar, carve out rounds into both slices of bread, remove the crusts.

Spread peanut butter evenly across one side of one of the rounds and spread jelly evenly across one side of the other round.

Place peanut butter round and jelly round together to create the "body" of the spider.

Place 4 pretzel sticks into the left side of the sandwich and 4 pretzel sticks into the right side, creating the "spider legs."

Place raisins on the sandwich to create the "eyes."

Enjoy!

Salted Honey Apple Brie Grilled Cheese

Ingredients

for 2 servings

4 slices fruit and nut bread, or rustic bread of choice

2 tablespoons unsalted butter, room temperature

2 tablespoons whole-grain Dijon mustard

1 granny smith apple, halved, cored, and sliced 1/8–1/4-inch-thick

2 teaspoons honey, plus more serving

flaky sea salt, for sprinkling

8 oz brie cheese (225 g), rind removed and sliced

Directions

Heat a large griddle or skillet over medium-low heat.

Spread the butter on one side of each slice of bread. Flip the bread over and spread the mustard on 2 slices, then layer the apple slices on top of the mustard. Drizzle the honey over the apples, then sprinkle with a pinch of flaky salt. Arrange the Brie on the other slices of bread. Close the sandwiches.

Transfer the sandwiches to the pan and cook until golden brown on each side and the cheese has melted, 7–9 minutes per side.

Remove the sandwiches from the pan and cut in half. Top with another drizzle of honey and a sprinkle of flaky salt. Serve immediately.

Enjoy!

Instant Pot Pulled Chicken

Ingredients

for 4 servings

1 whole chicken

2 teaspoons kosher salt

1 teaspoon freshly ground black pepper

1 tablespoon olive oil

1 cup low sodium chicken broth (240 mL)

½ cup barbecue sauce (120 g)

bun, for serving - optional

Directions

On a cutting board, pat the chicken dry with paper towels. Season all over with the salt and pepper.

Set the Instant Pot to sauté and add the olive oil. Once the oil begins to shimmer, add the chicken, breast side-down, and cook until golden brown, about 5 minutes. Flip the chicken over with tongs and continue to cook until golden brown on the other side, about 5 minutes more. Remove the chicken from the Instant Pot and transfer to a clean cutting board.

Place the trivet in the bottom of the Instant Pot and pour in the chicken broth. Place the chicken, breast side-up, on the trivet, and cover the pot. Set to manual pressure for 35 minutes. Once the timer is up, let the Instant Pot release naturally for 30 minutes.

Remove the chicken with tongs and transfer to a cutting board. Use 2 forks to shred the meat, then transfer to a medium bowl. Discard the skin and bones. Add the barbecue sauce and stir until combined.

Serve the chicken on the buns or as desired.

Enjoy!

Suugo Suqaar

Ingredients

for 6 servings

Xawaash Spice Mix

1 whole cinnamon stick

½ cup whole cumin seeds (55 g)

½ cup whole coriander seeds (40 g)

2 tablespoons whole black peppercorn

6 whole cardamom pods

1 teaspoon whole clove

2 teaspoons ground turmeric

Suugo Suqaar

3 tablespoons olive oil

2 cloves garlic, minced

1 small green bell pepper, seeded and finely diced

1 small red onion, finely diced

1 lb ground beef (425 g), 80/20

1 teaspoon kosher salt, plus more to taste

2 tablespoons tomato paste

1 can tomato, diced

For Serving

1 lb spaghetti (425 g), cooked according to package instructions

fresh cilantro leaf, minced

banana

Directions

Make the xawaash spice mix: Place the cinnamon stick in a small zip-top bag. Seal the bag and use a heavy skillet or rolling pin to smash the cinnamon stick into smaller pieces.

Transfer the cinnamon to a medium heavy-bottomed skillet and add the cumin, coriander, peppercorns, cardamom, cloves, and turmeric. Cook over medium heat, stirring constantly, until the spices are lightly toasted and very aromatic, about 2 minutes. Remove the pan from the heat and set aside to cool.

Once cooled, transfer the toasted spices to a clean spice grinder or mortar and pestle and grind into a fine powder. Sift the ground spices through a fine-mesh sieve into a medium airtight container. Grind any large pieces left behind in the sieve, then sift into the container.

Cover and store in a cool, dark place until ready to use, up to 6 months.

Make the suugo suqaar: Heat the olive oil in a large, high-walled skillet or Dutch oven over medium-high heat. Once the oil is shimmering, add the garlic, bell pepper, and onion. Cook, stirring occasionally, until the vegetables begin to soften, about 8 minutes. Add the beef, salt, and 3 tablespoons of the Xawaash spice mixture, and cook, stirring occasionally to break up the beef, until the meat is browned, about 15 minutes.

Add the tomato paste and diced tomatoes. Fill the tomato can halfway with water and add to the pan. Stir well to combine, being sure to scrape up any browned bits stuck to the bottom of the pan. Increase the heat to high and bring the sauce to a boil, then decrease the heat to low, cover, and simmer, stirring occasionally, for about 30 minutes, until the sauce is thickened and the beef is tender. Season with more salt to taste.

Serve the sauce hot over spaghetti, garnished with cilantro. Serve with fresh banana. Any leftover sauce will keep in an airtight container in the refrigerator for up to 4 days. Rewarm in a heavy pot over low heat.

Enjoy!

Instant Pot Beef Chili

Ingredients

for 4 servings

1 tablespoon olive oil

1 medium yellow onion, diced

3 cloves garlic, minced

1 jalapeño, seeded and minced

1 lb ground beef (455 g)

2 teaspoons kosher salt

1 teaspoon freshly ground black pepper

1 teaspoon ground cumin

1 teaspoon smoked paprika

1 teaspoon chili powder

¼ cup tomato paste (55 g)

1 can whole peeled tomato

1 can kidney bean, drained and rinsed

1 ½ cups chicken stock (360 mL)

shredded cheddar cheese, for serving

fresh cilantro, roughly chopped, for serving

sour cream, for serving

Directions

Set the Instant Pot to sauté and add the olive oil. Once the oil begins to shimmer, add the onion and cook, stirring often, until starting to soften, about 5 minutes. Add the garlic and jalapeño and cook, stirring frequently, until aromatic, 1 minute.

Add the ground beef and cook, breaking up with a wooden spoon, until browned and cooked through, about 7 minutes. Add the salt, pepper, cumin, paprika, chili powder, and tomato paste and cook, stirring constantly, until combined, 1 minute.

Add the tomatoes and use a potato masher to break up, then add the kidney beans and chicken stock. Place the lid on the Instant Pot and set to pressure cook on high for 20 minutes. Once the timer goes off, set the Instant Pot to quick release.

Serve the chili with shredded cheddar cheese, cilantro, and sour cream.

Enjoy!

Cacio E Pepe Pizza

Ingredients

for 1 pizza

Pizza Dough

2 cups bread flour (250 g), plus more for dusting

1 cup warm water (240 mL)

¾ teaspoon instant yeast

2 teaspoons kosher salt

2 tablespoons olive oil, divided

2 teaspoons crushed ice

Parmesan Cream

½ cup whole milk ricotta cheese (120 mL)

¼ cup freshly grated parmigiano-reggiano cheese (55 g)

2 tablespoons heavy cream

Assembly

8 slices fresh mozzarella cheese

1 cup shredded pecorino romano cheese (100 g)

1 tablespoon freshly ground black pepper

Directions

Make the pizza Dough: In a large bowl, combine the flour and warm water and stir with your hands until a shaggy mass forms (it will be a little dry, but will hydrate after resting). Cover the bowl with a kitchen towel and let the Dough rest at room temperature for 20 minutes.

Uncover the bowl and sprinkle the yeast and salt over the Dough. Stir with a wooden spoon until the yeast and salt are evenly distributed.

Turn the Dough out onto a lightly floured surface and knead until a smooth ball forms, about 10 minutes. It will be very sticky because of the high hydration. Try not to use too much extra flour; instead use a bench scraper or flat metal spatula to scrape the Dough from the surface and continue kneading. You can also dip your palms in flour to help keep the Dough from sticking.

Grease a clean large bowl with 1 tablespoon of olive oil, then place the Dough in the bowl, cover with the kitchen towel, and let rise in a warm place until doubled in size, about 90 minutes. Remove the towel and loosely cover the bowl with plastic wrap, then place in the refrigerator overnight.

Make the Parmesan cream: Add the ricotta, Parmigiano-Reggiano, and heavy cream to a blender and blend on medium speed until just combined, about 15 seconds. Transfer to a zip-top bag and refrigerate until ready to use.

Remove the Dough from the refrigerator and let come to room temperature, about 30 minutes.

Preheat the oven to 500°F (260°C). Place a baking sheet, upside down, in the center of the oven while it preheats.

Drizzle the remaining tablespoon of olive oil over a clean baking sheet.

Transfer the Dough from the bowl to the oiled baking sheet. Gently use your hands to stretch it into a 12-inch round. Place the crushed ice in the center of the Dough.

Place the baking sheet with the pizza in the oven on top of the inverted baking sheet. Bake until the edges begin to crisp and the pizza Dough is light golden in color, about 8 minutes.

Remove the pizza from the oven and arrange the mozzarella slices evenly on top, then sprinkle with the Pecorino Romano.

Return the pizza to the oven and continue baking until the cheese is completely melted, about 4 minutes more.

Remove the pizza from the oven and use a pepper mill to evenly grind the black pepper over the entire pizza.

Cut a ½-inch opening from the corner of the zip-top bag with the Parmesan cream, then drizzle in a circular pattern over the pizza.

Slice into 8 pieces and serve.

Enjoy!

Tandoori Turkey

Ingredients

for 12 servings

Tandoori Spice Blend

4 cinnamon sticks, broekn into 1in (2.54 cm) pieces

¼ cup whole coriander (10 g)

3 tablespoons whole cumin seeds

3 whole mace blades

1 ½ tablespoons whole fenugreek seeds

1 tablespoon whole black cardamom pod

1 tablespoon whole green cardamom pods

1 tablespoon whole black peppercorn

1 tablespoon whole clove

3 tablespoons kashmiri chile powder

1 tablespoon ground ginger

1 tablespoon garlic powder

2 teaspoons freshly grated nutmeg

Yogurt Marinade

32 oz plain full-fat greek yogurt (955 g)

¼ cup lemon juice (60 mL)

¼ cup kosher salt (30 g)

1 tablespoon grated fresh ginger

1 tablespoon grated garlic

Turkey

1 turkey, thawed

Tandoori Ghee

1 ½ cups ghee (325 g), clarified butter

2 teaspoons kosher salt

For Roasting

2 lemons, quartered

1 head garlic, halved crosswise

4 fresh bay leaves

1 piece fresh ginger, sliced into 1/2 in thick rounds

½ bunch fresh cilantro

3 cups chicken stock (720 mL)

Gravy

¼ cup all purpose flour (25 g), plus 2 tablespoons

3 cups reserved turkey drippings (720 mL), fat separated and discarded, warmed, or chicken stock

For Serving

fresh cilantro, chopped

lime, quartered

Traditional Tandoori side dish, such as rice pulao, raita, aaan, kachumber, and/or aloo bhaji

Directions

Make the tandoori spice blend: Set a medium skillet over medium-low heat and let the pan warm for a few minutes. Working one spice group at a time, toast the cinnamon sticks, coriander seeds, cumin seeds, mace blades (if using), fenugreek seeds, black and green cardamom pods, black peppercorns, and cloves in the warm skillet until each spice is fragrant and lightly browned, a few minutes per spice. Transfer the toasted spices to a plate or small tray while you toast the remaining spices. Let cool to room temperature.

Set a mesh strainer over a medium bowl. Once all of the whole spices have cooled, transfer to a high-powered blender or spice grinder (working in batches, if needed) and grind the spices into a fine powder. Pour the ground spices into the strainer and sift into the bowl below. Return any larger pieces to the blender and re-grind and sift into the bowl.

Add the Kashmiri chile powder, ground ginger, garlic powder, and nutmeg to the bowl with the ground spices and mix well to combine (if using ground mace, add here). Transfer the mixture to an airtight container and store in a cool, dry place until ready to use. The spice mixture will keep for up to 2 weeks.

Make the yogurt marinade: In a medium bowl, whisk together the yogurt, ¾ cup of the tandoori spice blend, the lemon juice, salt, ginger, and garlic until smooth.

Remove the innards from the turkey and discard (or save for another use). Pat the turkey dry all over with paper towels. Place the turkey in a bowl large enough to fit the bird, then pour the yogurt marinade all over the turkey. Use your fingers to gently loosen the turkey skin, starting from the top of the cavity and working your way toward the breasts and down toward the legs, being careful not to tear the skin. Use your hands to work the marinade underneath the skin and all over the entire bird. Once well-coated, cover the bowl with plastic wrap and refrigerate for at least 3 hours, preferably overnight.

While the turkey is marinating, make the tandoori ghee: Add the ghee to a small saucepan and cook over medium heat for 2–3 minutes, until hot. Add 2 tablespoons of the tandoori spice blend (it should sizzle lightly once it touches the ghee), then stir to incorporate and remove the pot from the heat. Stir in the salt. Transfer ¼ cup of the ghee to a small bowl and set aside to use for the gravy. Carefully pour the remaining 1¼ cups of ghee into a heat-proof container.

After marinating, remove the turkey from the refrigerator and let sit at room temperature for 2–3 hours before cooking.

Arrange a rack in the lower-middle section of the oven. Preheat the oven to 450°F (230°C). Set a V-shaped rack inside a roasting pan.

Once ready to cook, remove the turkey from the yogurt marinade and wipe off as much as possible. Squeeze out as much marinade as possible from underneath the turkey skin as well.

Grab the turkey by the legs and carefully transfer to the prepared roasting pan with the breast side up. With your hands, rub about a third of the tandoori ghee over the bird, then rub another third underneath the skin. Reserve the remaining ghee for basting the turkey.

Stuff the cavity with the lemons, garlic, ginger, and cilantro. Tuck the wings underneath the turkey, then tie the legs together with kitchen twine, wrapping around the bird to secure.

Pour 3 cups of chicken stock into the bottom of the roasting pan.

Roast the turkey for 30 minutes, rotating halfway, until the skin is mostly golden brown. While the turkey roasts, melt the remaining third of tandoori ghee in a small saucepan over low heat, or in a small bowl in the microwave.

After roasting for 30 minutes, baste the turkey with the melted ghee. Reduce the oven temperature to 300°F (150°C). If the bottom of the pan looks dry, pour in 1–2 more cups of stock. Continue roasting, basting and rotating the turkey every 30 minutes, until a meat thermometer inserted in the thickest part of the leg reaches 165°F (75°C), 120–150 minutes more. The skin should be shiny, crisp, and golden brown—if the skin begins to get too dark, lightly tend the bird with aluminum foil.

Remove the turkey from the oven and baste once more. Let rest for 30–60 minutes. Reserve the drippings, discarding the fat, for making the gravy.

Make the tandoori gravy: Add the reserved ¼ cup tandoori ghee to a medium saucepan over medium heat. Add the flour and cook, whisking frequently, for 3–5 minutes, until the roux is darker in color and smells fragrant and toasted. Add 1 tablespoon of the tandoori spice blend and whisk to combine, letting toast for another minute, until fragrant. Gradually whisk in the turkey drippings (adding chicken stock as needed for a total of 3 cups). Bring to a boil, then reduce the heat to medium-low and simmer for 10–15 minutes, until thickened slightly. Remove the gravy from heat.

To serve, set the whole turkey in the center of a large platter for a classic presentation, or carve the bird and arrange the cut pieces on the platter and garnish with cilantro and quartered limes. Serve immediately with the hot gravy alongside, as well as any traditional tandoori sides of choice.

Enjoy!

DINNER RECIPES SUGGESTIONS

Crunchy Avocado Tuna Wraps

Ingredients

for 4 servings

5 oz tuna (140 g), 2 cans, drained

1 large avocado, diced

1 cup carrot (110 g), finely chopped

2 ribs celery, finely chopped

¼ cup red onion (35 g), finely chopped

¼ cup dijon mustard (60 g)

1 tablespoon lemon juice

½ teaspoon garlic powder

salt, to taste

pepper, to taste

4 whole wheat tortillas

4 leaves green leaf lettuce

1 cup cherry tomatoes (200 g), halved

Directions

In a large bowl, add the tuna and avocado. Use a fork to smash the avocado and tuna together.

Add the carrots, celery, red onion, Dijon mustard, lemon juice, garlic powder, salt, and pepper. Stir to combine.

Lay a tortilla flat on a plate. Lay a lettuce leaf on the tortilla. Scoop ¼ of the tuna mixture into the center of the lettuce and spread down the middle. Top with cherry tomatoes and carefully roll the the tortilla to create a wrap. Repeat with the remaining Ingredients.

Enjoy!

Korean-Style BBQ Pork Ribs

Ingredients

for 2 servings

For the sauce:

3 tablespoons sesame oil

2 teaspoons rice wine vinegar

3 tablespoons dark soy sauce

4 tablespoons honey

30 mL bourbon whiskey (30 mL)

15 mL fresh lime juice (15 mL)

4 medium cloves garlic cloves, finely chopped

2 teaspoons smoked paprika

4 tablespoons dark muscovado sugar

1 teaspoon red chili flakes

2 teaspoons corn flour

1 teaspoon sesame seeds

For the ribs:

1 whole rack of pork ribs

For the rub:

1 tablespoon kosher salt

1 tablespoon pepper

1 tablespoon dark muscovado sugar

Directions

Preheat the oven to 150 degrees celsius.

Mix together the salt, pepper and sugar for the rub and apply liberally over the ribs.

Wrap entirely in foil and bake in the oven for 2 hours at 150 degrees celsius / 300 degrees Fahrenheit.

In a saucepan, combine all of the sauce Ingredientsand bring to a boil then immediately reduce the heat until the sauce thickens and then set aside.

Remove the ribs from the oven and unwrap from the foil. Brush a generous amount of the BBQ sauce over both sides of the ribs and place back in the oven for a further 10 minutes.

Remove from the oven, brush more bbq sauce on and sprinkle with sesame seeds.

Enjoy!

Pumpkin Sage Pasta

Ingredients

for 4 servings

1 tablespoon cooking oil, of preference

½ white onion, diced

2 cloves garlic, minced

½ teaspoon red pepper flakes, optional

½ teaspoon dried sage

1 ½ cups almond milk (360 mL)

15 oz pumpkin puree (425 g)

1 teaspoon salt

1 teaspoon pepper

¼ teaspoon nutmeg

½ box whole wheat pasta, cooked

Directions

Heat the oil in a medium pot over medium heat. Add the onion, garlic, red pepper flakes, and dried sage and cook until onions are translucent, stirring occasionally.

Add the almond milk, pumpkin puree, salt, pepper, and nutmeg. Stir until a smooth, creamy sauce forms. Heat through.

Add the cooked pasta and and stir to coat.

Serve warm.

Enjoy!

One-Pan Chicken Adobo

Ingredients

for 4 servings

2 lb chicken (910 g)

3 dried bay leaves

5 tablespoons soy sauce

2 tablespoons vinegar

3 garlics, crushed

1 cup water (240 mL)

¼ cup cooking oil (60 mL)

1 tablespoon white sugar

salt, to taste

whole peppercorn

Directions

In a container or a plastic food bag, combine soy sauce and garlic then marinade the chicken for 30 minutes.

Place a medium pan on medium heat and add oil, once the oil is hot put the marinated chicken and brown (about five minutes).

Pour in the remaining marinade and add water, then bring to a boil.

Add the dried bay leaves and whole peppercorn. Simmer for 30 minutes or until the chicken is tender.

Add the vinegar, stir and simmer for 10 more minutes.

Add the sugar, salt, and stir. Then remove from heat.

Enjoy!

Whole-roasted Chicken and Veggies

Ingredients

for 6 servings

2 carrots, diced

1 cup butternut squash (125 g), diced

1 ½ cups broccoli floret (225 g)

2 tablespoons oil

4 lb small whole chicken (2 kg)

salt, to taste

black pepper, to taste

1 leaf fresh thyme leaf, to taste

3 sprigs fresh thyme sprigs, for garnish

butcher's twine

Directions

Preheat oven to 425°F (220°C).

In a large, ovenproof skillet or frying pan, mix together the carrots, squash, and broccoli, and coat with the oil. Spread the veggies into 1 even layer.

Place the chicken on top of the veggies.

Season the bird on all sides and in the cavity with salt, pepper, and fresh thyme leaves. While seasoning the bird, make sure that enough seasoning has fallen onto the veggies below to give them good flavor.

To truss the chicken, fold the wingtips underneath the breasts so that they fit snugly. Using a piece of butcher's twine, tie the legs together so the bird holds a nice shape.

Bake for 1 hour, or until a thermometer inserted into the thickest part of the breast reads 160°F (70°C).

NOTE: Once resting out of the oven, the temperature will continue to rise to a safe 165°F (75°C).

Let the chicken rest for at least 15 minutes once out of the oven, so that all of the juices in the meat can settle and the internal temperature has time to finish rising.

Carve the bird as desired.

Serve on a plate with the veggies, and fresh thyme sprigs for garnish.

Enjoy!

One-Pan Whole Roasted Chicken & Veggies

Ingredients

for 6 servings

1 medium yellow onion, thinly sliced

6 medium carrots, cut on the bias into 1/2 inch (12MM) slices

1 package tuscan kale, about 1/2 bunch, stem removed

3 tablespoons extra virgin olive oil, divided

kosher salt, to taste

black pepper, to taste

½ cup white wine (120 mL), such as Pinot Grigio or Sauvignon Blanc

3 lb whole chicken (1.5 kg), giblets removed, patted dry

8 sprigs fresh rosemary

8 sprigs fresh thyme

1 lemon, halved

Special Equipment

cast iron pan, 12 inch (30 cm)

kitchen twine

Directions

Arrange an oven rack in the center of the oven, then preheat to 425°F (220°C).

Toss the onion, carrots, and kale in a 12-inch (30 cm) cast iron skillet with 2 tablespoons of olive oil, salt, and pepper until well coated. Pour the white wine over the vegetables.

Season the chicken all over with salt and pepper, then brush with the remaining tablespoon of olive oil. Stuff the rosemary, thyme, and lemon inside the cavity, tie the legs closed with kitchen twine, and tuck the wings underneath the bird. Place the chicken, breast-side up, on top of the vegetables in the skillet.

Roast the chicken for 1 hour, rotating the pan halfway through cooking. The chicken is done when it is golden brown, the skin is crispy, and an instant-read thermometer inserted into the thigh registers 165°F (70°C). Remove from the oven and let the chicken rest for 15 minutes.

Carve the chicken, then plate alongside the vegetables. Pour the pan drippings over the top and serve immediately.

Enjoy!

Tuna Burgers

Ingredients

for 4 servings

15 oz tuna (425 g), canned, drained

1 tablespoon olive oil, plus more for cooking

¾ cup panko bread crumbs (35 g)

1 tablespoon dried parsley

2 teaspoons fresh chives, minced

1 tablespoon garlic, minced

½ teaspoon salt

½ teaspoon pepper

1 teaspoon paprika

1 large egg, beaten

whole wheat burger bun, for serving

Directions

Combine the tuna, olive oil, panko, parsley, chives, garlic, salt, pepper, paprika, and egg in a large bowl until evenly mixed.

Divide the mixture into 4 portions and form patties with your hands.

Heat a drizzle of olive oil in a large skillet over medium-high heat.

Place the patties in the pan and cook for 3-5 minutes on each side, until golden brown.

Serve on whole wheat buns with your preferred toppings.

Enjoy!

Pesto Garden Pasta For The Whole Family

Ingredients

for 6 servings

Pesto Sauce

2 cups fresh basil leaves (80 g)

½ cup olive oil (120 mL)

½ cup grated parmesan cheese (55 g)

1 tablespoon almond butter

1 tablespoon lemon juice

2 cloves garlic, smashed

2 teaspoons lemon zest

kosher salt, to taste

pepper, to taste

Pasta

kosher salt, to taste

4 cups pasta (800 g), short, such as farfalle or penne

1 cup grape tomato (200 g), halved

1 cup yellow cherry tomato (200 g), halved

¼ cup red onion (35 g), sliced

8 oz mozzarella ball (225 g), drained

Directions

Add the basil, olive oil, Parmesan, almond butter, lemon juice, garlic, lemon zest, salt, and pepper to a blender. Blend until smooth and set aside.

Cook the pasta according to the package instructions.

Drain and transfer the pasta to a large serving bowl.

Add the grape tomatoes, yellow tomatoes, red onion, and mozzarella balls to the pasta.

Pour the pesto sauce over the pasta.

Toss the Ingredients together.

Serve warm in a bowl.

Enjoy!

Instant-Pot Whole Herb Chicken

Ingredients

for 6 servings

1 tablespoon fresh sage, minced

1 tablespoon fresh thyme, minced

1 tablespoon fresh chives, plus more for garnish

¼ cup oil (60 mL), divided, plus 1 tablespoon

kosher salt, to taste

3 ½ lb whole chicken (1.5 kg), rinsed and patted dry

ground black pepper, to taste

3 lemons, quartered and seeded, divided

1 medium yellow onion, roughly chopped

4 cloves garlic, smashed

1 ½ cups chicken stock (360 mL)

½ cup dry sherry (120 mL)

3 tablespoons water

3 tablespoons cornstarch

Directions

In a small bowl, combine the sage, thyme, chives, ¼ cup (60 ML) oil, and a pinch of salt. Stir into a paste. Set aside.

Generously season the chicken all over with salt and pepper. Then, using your fingers, gently release the skin over the chicken breast so that your fingers can slide between the skin and the breast meat. Spread half of the herb paste evenly between both breasts, then massage the skin with your fingers to push the herb paste to the places it didn't reach. Reserve the remaining herb paste for later. Place 1 quartered lemon inside the cavity, then tie the legs together with kitchen twine. Tuck the wings under the chicken.

To a 6-quart Instant-Pot, add the onion, remaining 2 lemons, and the garlic. Place the chicken, breast-side up, on top, then pour in the chicken stock and sherry. Brush the remaining herb paste over the chicken. Cover with the Instant Pot lid, making sure the release valve is set to "sealing." Set the Instant Pot to high pressure cook for 25 minutes.

Release the pressure from the Instant Pot by switching the vent from "sealing" to "venting," making sure your hand is not over the top of the release switch, as the hot steam will come out of the top. Wait for the pressure to release and the Instant Pot to unlock before taking off the lid.

Transfer the chicken from the Instant Pot onto a baking sheet. If you would like crispier skin, set the broiler to high. Roast the chicken under the broiler for 3-4 minutes, or until the skin crisps and becomes a deep golden brown.

While the chicken skin crisps, turn the Instant Pot to high sauté mode. Bring the liquid in the pot to a boil and reduce by half, 5-6 minutes.

Add the cornstarch to the water and whisk together until smooth. When the sauce is reduced, whisk in the cornstarch slurry and continue to boil the gravy for another 2 minutes, or until the gravy is thick and coats the back of a spoon.

Strain the gravy through a fine mesh sieve.

Cut the chicken off the bone, place on a platter, and garnish with chives. Serve with the gravy.

Enjoy!

Country Fried Steak And Gravy

Ingredients

for 4 servings

8 oz cube steak (225 g), 4 steaks, 8 oz (225 g) each

1 ½ teaspoons kosher salt, plus more to taste

1 teaspoon black pepper, plus more to taste

2 large eggs

2 ¾ cups whole milk (660 mL), divided

1 ½ cups all-purpose flour (190 g), divided, plus 3 tablespoons

1 teaspoon garlic powder

1 teaspoon onion powder

1 teaspoon paprika

1 cup vegetable oil (240 mL)

3 tablespoons unsalted butter

½ cup heavy cream (120 mL)

Directions

Preheat the oven to 225°F (110°C).

Set a steak in the center of a cutting board and cover with a piece of plastic wrap. Using a meat mallet, pound the steak evenly to ¼-inch (½ cm) thick. Season with salt and pepper on both sides. Repeat with the remaining meat.

In a wide, shallow dish, whisk together the eggs and 1 cup (240 ml) of milk. In a separate shallow dish, mix together the 1 ½ cups (190 g) of flour, pepper, salt, garlic powder, onion powder, and paprika.

Dredge the steaks in the flour mixture, then dip in the egg mixture, letting any excess egg drip off. Coat again in the flour mixture. Set aside for 10-15 minutes, until the coating has dried out a bit.

Meanwhile, heat the oil in a 10-inch (25.5 cm) pan over medium-high heat until it reaches $375\,^\circ\text{F}$ ($190\,^\circ\text{C}$).

Fry the steaks, 2 at a time, for 3 minutes, until golden brown and crispy. Flip and cook on the other side for 3 minutes more, until golden brown and cooked through when the internal temperature reaches $155\,^\circ$-$165\,^\circ\text{F}$ ($170\,^\circ$-$175\,^\circ\text{C}$).

Transfer the steaks to a paper towel-lined plate or baking sheet and immediately season with salt. Once all of the steaks are done frying, transfer to the oven while you prepare the gravy.

Pour the hot oil into a heatproof bowl and let cool before discarding. 9. Leave any browned bits in the pan.

In the same pan, without wiping it out, melt the butter over medium heat. Add the remaining 3 tablespoons of flour, whisking to incorporate. Cook for 2-3 minutes, until the roux is a light brown color. Add the heavy cream and remaining milk. Bring to a simmer and cook, whisking constantly, until thickened, 5-7 minutes. Season with salt and pepper.

Ladle the gravy over the steaks and serve with your favorite side dishes.

Enjoy!

One-Pot Cheesy Taco Pasta

Ingredients

for 10 servings

1 lb ground beef (455 g)

1 can tomato, diced (15 oz - 425g)

1 can whole kernel corn, (15 oz - 425g)

1 can tomato sauce, (15 oz - 425g)

2 cups water (480 mL)

1 package taco seasoning

salt, to taste

pepper, to taste

2 cups elbow macaroni (200 g), uncooked

1 ½ cups colby jack cheese (150 g)

Directions

In a large quart pot over medium-high heat brown the ground beef. Drain fat and return beef to the pot.

Add taco seasoning, water, diced tomatoes, corn and tomato sauce. Bring to a boil.

Add uncooked macaroni and reduce heat to low. Cover and simmer for 10-15 minutes (until pasta is cooked through). Stir occasionally.

Remove from heat. Sprinkle cheese on top and cover.

Serve once cheese is melted!

Enjoy!

BBQ Chicken Pita Pizza

Ingredients

for 1 serving

1 cup rotisserie chicken (125 g), shredded

⅛ cup BBQ sauce (30 g), + 2 tablespoons

1 whole wheat pita bread

1 handful shredded mozzarella cheese

1 handful red onion, sliced

fresh cilantro, for garnish

Directions

Preheat oven to 350°F (180°C).

In a small bowl, combine chicken and bbq sauce well. Set aside.

Place pita bread on a baking sheet lined with parchment and spread bbq sauce over it.

Add the chicken to the pita and sprinkle with mozzarella and red onion, to taste.

Bake for 15-20 minutes, or until cheese is melted and chicken is heated through.

Garnish with fresh cilantro, slice, and serve.

Enjoy!

Veggie-Packed Chicken Enchiladas

Ingredients

for 6 servings

2 cups tomato sauce (520 g)

1 cup vegetable broth (240 mL)

salt, to taste

pepper, to taste

¼ teaspoon chile powder

¼ teaspoon cumin

¼ teaspoon garlic powder

2 medium zucchinis

½ red onion, diced

2 boneless, skinless chicken breasts, cooked and shredded

6 medium whole wheat tortillas

2 cups shredded cheese (200 g)

fresh cilantro, to serve, optional

Directions

Preheat oven to 400°F (200°C).

In a medium saucepan over medium heat, add the tomato sauce, vegetable broth, salt, pepper, chile powder, cumin and garlic powder.

Stir occasionally, until the sauce begins to boil. Remove from the heat.

Using a box grater, grate the zucchini.

In a large skillet over medium heat, add grated zucchini, red onion, salt and pepper. Cook until onions are translucent.

Add chicken and ¼ of the tomato sauce mixture. Combine well and remove from heat.

Fill the tortillas with the zucchini mixture and add cheese. Fold the tortillas over and place seam-side down into a greased baking dish. Repeat with remaining tortillas.

Pour the remaining tomato sauce over the tortillas and sprinkle with cheese.

Bake for 20 minutes, or until heated through and cheese is melted.

Top with cilantro (optional).

Enjoy!

Sun-Dried Tomato & Spinach Tuna Pasta

Ingredients

for 2 servings

1 tablespoon olive oil

1 tablespoon garlic, minced

½ cup sundried tomato (25 g)

1 lemon, juiced

10 oz tuna (285 g), canned, drained

salt, to taste

pepper, to taste

2 cups whole wheat pasta (200 g), cooked according to package instructions

2 cups fresh spinach (80 g)

Directions

Heat the olive oil in a large skillet over medium-high heat. Add the garlic and cook for about 30 seconds, until fragrant.

Add the sun-dried tomatoes and lemon juice and cook for 1-2 minutes, until fragrant.

Add the tuna, salt, and pepper, and mix until thoroughly combined.

Add the pasta and spinach and cook for about 1 minute, until spinach starts to wilt.

Remove the pasta from the heat and serve.

Enjoy!

Audrey Hepburn's Spaghetti Al Pomodoro

Ingredients

for 4 servings

2 tablespoons extra virgin olive oil

1 whole small onion, diced

2 stalks celery, finely diced

2 cloves garlic, minced

1 large bunch fresh basil, washed, half of the leaves minced and half left whole

28 oz canned whole peeled tomato (795 g), 2 cans

salt, to taste

1 lb dried spathetti (455 g)

½ cup freshly grated parmigiano-reggiano cheese (55 g)

1 cup carrots (125 g), diced

Directions

Dice the carrots, onion, and celery. Thinly slice half of the basil leaves. Set aside.

Heat the olive oil in a large pot over medium heat. Add the onion, carrots, celery, and garlic. Cook until softened but not brown.

Add in the whole basil leaves, garlic, and tomatoes. Bring the sauce to a simmer, cover, and cook for 45 minutes, stirring occasionally and breaking apart the larger tomatoes as they cook.

After 45 minutes, or when the vegetables are tender, remove the sauce from the heat and let rest for 15 minutes.

While the sauce is simmering, fill another large pot with water and bring to a boil. Add salt, if desired. Cook the spaghetti until al dente. Drain and rinse the pasta with lukewarm water to prevent sticking.

Taste the sauce and add salt, if desired. Serve pasta topped generously with sauce, grated Parmigiano-Reggiano cheese, and the reserved sliced basil leaves.

Enjoy!

Elevated Hamburger Helper

Ingredients

for 4 servings

8 oz bacon (225 g), chopped

1 small yellow onion, chopped

½ cup red bell pepper (50 g), minced

1 cup shredded carrot (100 g)

2 cloves garlic, grated

1 lb lean ground beef (425 g)

kosher salt, to taste

1 tablespoon smoked paprika

2 tablespoons tomato paste, preferable double-concentrated

1 can diced tomato, petite

3 cups beef stock (720 mL)

2 cups whole milk (480 mL)

1 lb pasta shells (425 g), or short noodles of choice

2 cups shredded smoked gouda cheese (200 g)

2 cups shredded cheddar cheese (200 g)

fresh parsley, for garnish

Directions

Add the bacon to a large pot. Turn the heat to medium-high and cook until crispy, 5–7 minutes. Using a slotted spoon, transfer the bacon to a paper towel-lined plate to drain. Discard all but 1 tablespoon of the rendered bacon fat in the pot.

Reduce the heat to medium and add the onion to the pot. Cook until softened, 5–7 minutes. Add the red bell pepper, carrots, and garlic. Cook until softened, 2–3 minutes more.

Increase the heat to medium-high and add the ground beef to the pan. Break up the beef with spatula and cook until browned, about 5 minutes. Season with salt.

Add the paprika and tomato paste. Cook until fragrant and the tomato paste turns brick-red in color, 2–3 minutes. Add the diced tomatoes, beef stock, and milk and bring to a low boil.

Once the liquid is boiling, add the pasta shells. Cover and cook for about 10 minutes, stirring occasionally, until the noodles are al dente and they have absorbed most of the liquid. NOTE: The timing will differ depending on what type of noodles you use.

Remove the pot from the heat. Stir in the Gouda and cheddar cheeses until melted. Fold in the cooked bacon.

Garnish with parsley, if desired.

Serve immediately.

Enjoy!

SECTION 5: IN SUMMARY!

The journey through understanding and managing angioedema through dietary modifications is both empowering and enlightening. The Angioedema Diet offers not just a collection of recipes, but a comprehensive guide to navigating the complexities of this condition. By embracing the principles of inflammation reduction, immune system support, and allergen avoidance, individuals can embark on a path towards improved health and well-being.

Throughout this book, we have explored the intricate relationship between food and angioedema, uncovering the potential triggers and culprits behind swelling episodes. Armed with knowledge and practical advice, readers are equipped to make informed choices that support their unique dietary needs and preferences while mitigating the risks associated with this condition.

Moreover, the journey doesn't end here. It is a continuous process of self-discovery and adaptation, where individuals learn to listen to their bodies, recognize patterns, and fine-tune their dietary approach accordingly. With each step forward, individuals gain greater control over their health and find relief from the burdens of angioedema.

As we close this chapter, let us remember that the Angioedema Diet is not just about what we eat, but about nourishing our bodies, minds, and spirits. It is a journey of resilience, hope, and empowerment—a journey towards a life filled with vitality and well-being.